# Gastrointestinal Issues in Critical Care

*Editors*

RAHUL S. NANCHAL
RAM M. SUBRAMANIAN

# CRITICAL CARE CLINICS

www.criticalcare.theclinics.com

*Consulting Editor*
RICHARD W. CARLSON

April 2016 • Volume 32 • Number 2

**ELSEVIER**

1600 John F. Kennedy Boulevard • Suite 1800 • Philadelphia, Pennsylvania, 19103-2899

http://www.theclinics.com

**CRITICAL CARE CLINICS Volume 32, Number 2**
**April 2016 ISSN 0749-0704, ISBN-13: 978-0-323-41748-8**

Editor: Patrick Manley
Developmental Editor: Casey Jackson



*Critical Care Clinics* (ISSN: 0749-0704) is published quarterly by Elsevier Inc., 360 Park Avenue South, New York, NY 10010-1710. Months of issue are January, April, July, and October. Business and Editorial Offices: 1600 John F. Kennedy Blvd., Suite 1800, Philadelphia, PA 19103-2899. Customer Service Office: 6277 Sea Harbor Drive, Orlando, FL 32887-4800. Periodicals postage paid at New York, NY and additional mailing offices. Subscription prices are $215.00 per year for US individuals, $551.00 per year for US institution, $100.00 per year for US students and residents, $255.00 per year for Canadian individuals, $691.00 per year for Canadian institutions, $300.00 per year for international individuals, $691.00 per year for international institutions and $150.00 per year for Canadian and foreign students/residents. To receive student/resident rate, orders must be accompanied by name of affiliated institution, date of term, and the signature of program/residency coordinator on institution letterhead. Orders will be billed at individual rate until proof of status is received. Foreign air speed delivery is included in all *Clinics* subscription prices. All prices are subject to change without notice. POSTMASTER: Send address changes to *Critical Care Clinics*, Elsevier Periodicals Customer Service, 11830 Westline Industrial Drive, St. Louis, MO 63146. **Customer Service: 1-800-654-2452 (US). From outside of the US, call 1-314-447-8871. Fax: 1-314-447-8029. E-mail: journalscustomerservice-usa@elsevier.com (for print support) or journalsonlinesupport-usa@elsevier.com (for online support).**

*Reprints*. For copies of 100 or more of articles in this publication, please contact the Commercial Reprints Department, Elsevier Inc., 360 Park Avenue South, New York, NY 10010-1710. Tel.: 212-633-3874; Fax: 212-633-3820; E-mail: reprints@elsevier.com.

*Critical Care Clinics* is also published in Spanish by Editorial Inter-Medica, Junin 917, 1er A, 1113, Buenos Aires, Argentina.

*Critical Care Clinics* is covered in *MEDLINE/PubMed (Index Medicus), EMBASE/Excerpta Medica, Current Concepts/Clinical Medicine, ISI/BIOMED, and Chemical Abstracts.*

# Contributors


## CONSULTING EDITOR

**RICHARD W. CARLSON, MD, PhD**
Chairman Emeritus, Director, Medical Intensive Care Unit, Department of Medicine, Maricopa Medical Center; Professor, University of Arizona College of Medicine; Professor, Department of Medicine, Mayo Graduate School of Medicine, Phoenix, Arizona; Mayo Clinic, Scottsdale, Arizona

## EDITORS

**RAHUL S. NANCHAL, MD, MS**
Associate Professor of Medicine and Neurology; Director, Critical Care Fellowship Program; Director, Medical Intensive Care Unit, Division of Pulmonary and Critical Care Medicine, Froedtert Health and Medical College of Wisconsin, Milwaukee, Wisconsin

**RAM M. SUBRAMANIAN, MD**
Associate Professor of Medicine and Surgery; Medical Director, Liver Transplantation, Emory University; Critical Care and Hepatology, Emory University School of Medicine, Atlanta, Georgia

## AUTHORS

**MARSHALL BECKMAN, MD**
Division of Trauma Surgery and Critical Care, Department of Surgery, Medical College of Wisconsin, Milwaukee, Wisconsin

**THOMAS W. CARVER, MD**
Associate Professor, Division of Trauma and Critical Care, Medical College of Wisconsin, Milwaukee, Wisconsin

**PANNA CODNER, MD**
Associate Professor, Division of Trauma and Acute Care Surgery, Department of Surgery, Medical College of Wisconsin, Milwaukee, Wisconsin

**CRAIG M. COOPERSMITH, MD**
Professor, Department of Surgery, Emory Critical Care Center, Emory University School of Medicine, Atlanta, Georgia

**GAURAV DAGAR, MD**
Assistant Professor of Medicine, Division of Pulmonary and Critical Care Medicine, Medical College of Wisconsin, Milwaukee, Wisconsin

**NATHAN J. KLINGENSMITH, MD**
Department of Surgery, Emory Critical Care Center, Emory University School of Medicine, Atlanta, Georgia

**RAHUL MAHESHWARI, MD**
Gastroenterology Fellow, Division of Digestive Diseases, Emory University School of Medicine, Atlanta, Georgia

**PATRICK MALUSO, MD**
Resident, Department of Surgery, George Washington University, Washington, DC

**RAHUL S. NANCHAL, MD, MS**
Associate Professor of Medicine and Neurology; Director, Critical Care Fellowship Program; Director, Medical Intensive Care Unit, Division of Pulmonary and Critical Care Medicine, Froedtert Health and Medical College of Wisconsin, Milwaukee, Wisconsin

**TODD NEIDEEN, MD**
Division of Trauma Surgery and Critical Care, Department of Surgery, Medical College of Wisconsin, Milwaukee, Wisconsin

**JODY OLSON, MD**
Assistant Professor of Medicine, Divisions of Hepatology and Liver Transplantation, University of Kansas, Kansas City, Kansas

**JAYSHIL J. PATEL, MD**
Assistant Professor, Division of Pulmonary and Critical Care Medicine, Department of Medicine, Medical College of Wisconsin, Milwaukee, Wisconsin

**JASMEET PAUL, MD**
Division of Trauma Surgery and Critical Care, Department of Surgery, Medical College of Wisconsin, Milwaukee, Wisconsin

**EMAD QAYED, MD**
Interim Chief of Gastroenterology, Grady Memorial Hospital; Assistant Professor of Medicine, Emory University School of Medicine, Atlanta, Georgia

**SYED IRFAN-UR RAHMAN, MD**
Resident, Department of Medicine, Medical College of Wisconsin, Milwaukee, Wisconsin

**KIA SAEIAN, MD, MSc Epi**
Associate Chief, Director of Clinical Affairs, Division of Gastroenterology and Hepatology, Department of Medicine, Medical College of Wisconsin, Milwaukee, Wisconsin

**BABAK SARANI, MD**
Associate Professor of Surgery, Department of Surgery; Director, Center for Trauma and Critical Care, George Washington University, Washington, DC

**RAM M. SUBRAMANIAN, MD**
Associate Professor of Medicine and Surgery; Medical Director, Liver Transplantation, Emory University; Critical Care and Hepatology, Emory University School of Medicine, Atlanta, Georgia

**AMIT TANEJA, MD**
Assistant Professor of Medicine, Division of Pulmonary and Critical Care Medicine, The Medical College of Wisconsin, Milwaukee, Wisconsin

**ROBERT W. TAYLOR, MD, MCCM**
Chairman, Department of Critical Care Medicine, Mercy Hospital St. Louis, St Louis, Missouri

**RAVI S. VORA, MD**
Fellow, Division of Digestive Diseases, Emory University, Atlanta, Georgia

**JOHN A. WEIGELT, MD, DVM**
Division of Trauma Surgery and Critical Care, Department of Surgery, Medical College of Wisconsin, Milwaukee, Wisconsin

# Contents

**Preface: Gastrointestinal Issues in Critical Care** xi

Rahul S. Nanchal and Ram M. Subramanian

**Mesenteric Ischemia** 155

Thomas W. Carver, Ravi S. Vora, and Amit Taneja

Acute mesenteric ischemia (AMI) is a rare disease that most commonly affects the elderly. The vague symptoms often lead to delayed diagnosis and consequent high mortality. Physical exam and laboratory findings lack the sensitivity and specificity to exclude AMI, but computed tomography angiography can rapidly and accurately confirm the diagnosis. Survival improves with prompt restoration of perfusion and resection of nonviable bowel. Advances in imaging, operative techniques, and critical care have led to a steady decline in overall mortality; however, long-term survival is limited because of the comorbidities in this patient group.

**Controversies in Critical Care Nutrition Support** 173

Jayshil J. Patel and Panna Codner

Critical illness predisposes individuals to highly variable metabolic and immune responses, leading to muscle mass loss, impaired healing, immobility, and susceptibility to infections and cognitive impairment. Recommendations for nutrition in critically ill patients are supported by observational studies, small randomized controlled trials, and mechanistic data. There is no standardization of nutritional therapy in critically ill patients and controversies in the type, quantity, and timing of nutrition support persist. This article reviews the physiologic basis for nutrition support, the concept of nutritional risk, and various controversies in critical care nutrition support.

**Gut Motility Issues in Critical Illness** 191

Robert W. Taylor

Acute gastrointestinal injury (AGI) is common in critical illness and negatively affects outcome. A variety of definitions have been used to describe AGI, which has led to clinical confusion and hampered comparison of research studies across institutions. An international working group of the European Society of Intensive Care Medicine was convened to standardize definitions for AGI and provide current evidence-based understanding of its pathophysiology and management. This disorder is associated with a wide variety of signs and symptoms and may be difficult to detect, therefore a high index of suspicion is warranted.

**The Gut as the Motor of Multiple Organ Dysfunction in Critical Illness** 203

Nathan J. Klingensmith and Craig M. Coopersmith

All elements of the gut - the epithelium, the immune system, and the microbiome - are impacted by critical illness and can, in turn, propagate a

pathologic host response leading to multiple organ dysfunction syndrome. Preclinical studies have demonstrated that this can occur by release of toxic gut-derived substances into the mesenteric lymph where they can cause distant damage. Further, intestinal integrity is compromised in critical illness with increases in apoptosis and permeability. There is also increasing recognition that microbes alter their behavior and can become virulent based upon host environmental cues. Gut failure is common in critically ill patients; however, therapeutics targeting the gut have proven to be challenging to implement at the bedside. Numerous strategies to manipulate the microbiome have recently been used with varying success in the ICU.

**Abdominal Compartment Hypertension and Abdominal Compartment Syndrome** **213**

Patrick Maluso, Jody Olson, and Babak Sarani

Intra-abdominal hypertension (IAH) and abdominal compartment syndrome (ACS) are rare but potentially morbid diagnoses. Clinical index of suspicion for these disorders should be raised following massive resuscitation, abdominal wall reconstruction/injury, and in those with space-occupying disorders in the abdomen. Gold standard for diagnosis involves measurement of bladder pressure, with a pressure greater than 12 mm Hg being consistent with IAH and greater than 25 mm Hg being consistent with ACS. Decompressive laparotomy is definitive therapy but paracentesis can be equally therapeutic in properly selected patients. Left untreated, ACS can lead to multisystem organ failure and death.

**Nonvariceal Upper Gastrointestinal Bleeding** **223**

Syed Irfan-Ur Rahman and Kia Saeian

In the intensive care unit, vigilance is needed to manage nonvariceal upper gastrointestinal bleeding. A focused history and physical examination must be completed to identify inciting factors and the need for hemodynamic stabilization. Although not universally used, risk stratification tools such as the Blatchford and Rockall scores can facilitate triage and management. Urgent evaluation for nonvariceal upper gastrointestinal bleeds requires prompt respiratory assessment, and identification of hemodynamic instability with fluid resuscitation and blood transfusions if necessary. Future studies are needed to evaluate the indication, safety, and efficacy of emerging endoscopic techniques.

**Lower Gastrointestinal Hemorrhage** **241**

Emad Qayed, Gaurav Dagar, and Rahul S. Nanchal

Lower gastrointestinal bleeding (LGIB) is a frequent reason for hospitalization especially in the elderly. Patients with LGIB are frequently admitted to the intensive care unit and may require transfusion of packed red blood cells and other blood products especially in the setting of coagulopathy. Colonoscopy is often performed to localize the source of bleeding and to provide therapeutic measures. LGIB may present as an acute life-threatening event or as a chronic insidious condition manifesting as iron deficiency anemia and positivity for fecal occult blood. This article

*Gastrointestinal Issues in Critical Care*

# CRITICAL CARE CLINICS

**FORTHCOMING ISSUES**

***July 2016***
**Hepatology and Critical Care**
Rahul Nanchal and Ram Subramaniam, *Editors*

***October 2016***
**Burn Resuscitation**
Daniel Caruso, Kevin Foster, and Michael Peck, *Editors*

***January 2017***
**Advances in Trauma**
Lena M. Napolitano, *Editor*

**RECENT ISSUES**

***January 2016***
**Obstetric and Gynecologic Emergencies**
Peter Papadakos and Susan Dantoni, *Editors*

***October 2015***
**Nephrology**
John Kellum, *Editor*

***July 2015***
**Sleep and Circadian Rhythms in the ICU**
Vipin Malik, *Editor*

**ISSUE OF RELATED INTEREST**

*Gastroenterology Clinics*, December 2014 (Vol. 43, No 4)
**Upper Gastrointestinal Bleeding**
Ian M. Gralnek, *Editor*

# Preface
# Gastrointestinal Issues in Critical Care

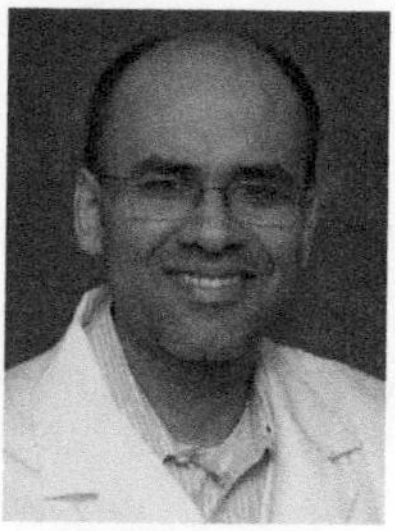
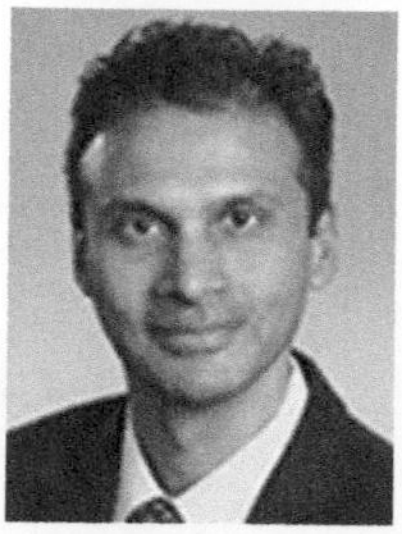

Rahul S. Nanchal, MD, MS   Ram M. Subramanian, MD
*Editors*

Hippocrates in 400 BC believed that "death sits in the bowel." The origins of the word sepsis derive from the verb form "sepo," which means "I rot." Hippocrates used the word to denote a state of odiferous biological decay and thought that this emanated from the colon, releasing "dangerous principles" and causing "auto-intoxication." Enemas ("physic") to cleanse the colon were thought to have immense medicinal value. Enemas were often given by the patient's caregivers, giving rise to the word "physician," or one who administers an enema. Leonardo da Vinci believed that the functions of the digestive system and respiratory system were interconnected. These historical descriptions are remarkably reminiscent of current paradigms, including "the gut motor hypothesis of multiple organ failure," gastrointestinal failure in critical illness, intra-abdominal hypertension, selective decontamination of the digestive tract, and the complex ways in which the abdomen influences systemic physiology. They also resonate with the exponentially expanding knowledge and armamentarium of emerging therapies related to the gastrointestinal system in critical illness.

Yet, in clinical practice, the importance of the gastrointestinal system and its influence on organ function in critical illness is poorly understood and often overlooked. Commonly used medications in intensive care units have profound implications on gut function. Abdominal pressure swings can incisively affect circulatory physiology. Research into the nuances of timing, route, and optimal dose of nutritional therapy in critical illness has created controversy and sparked intense debate but, more importantly, has furthered our understanding of the "gut in critical illness." In this issue, we have attempted to cover lacunae, answer a few questions, and elucidate principles that we believe are common dilemmas for the practicing intensivist.

A chance encounter many years ago set into motion a steadfast friendship and ever-growing productivity. To our wives, Nandita and Chinmayee, for their tireless

Crit Care Clin 32 (2016) xi–xii
http://dx.doi.org/10.1016/j.ccc.2016.01.001
0749-0704/16/$ – see front matter 

encouragement and unwavering patience, and to our children, Avi, Sanath, and Saurav, who make it possible for us to do what we do!

Rahul S. Nanchal, MD, MS
Medical Intensive Care Unit
Critical Care Fellowship Program
Froedtert Health and Medical College of Wisconsin
Milwaukee, WI 53226, USA

Ram M. Subramanian, MD
Emory University
Atlanta, GA 30322, USA

E-mail addresses:
Rnanchal@mcw.edu (R.S. Nanchal)
rmsubra@emory.edu (R.M. Subramanian)

# Mesenteric Ischemia

Thomas W. Carver, MD[a,*], Ravi S. Vora, MD[b], Amit Taneja, MD[c]

**KEYWORDS**

- Acute mesenteric ischemia • Nonocclusive mesenteric ischemia
- Arterial thrombosis • Mesenteric venous thrombosis • Mesenteric artery occlusion

**KEY POINTS**

- Acute mesenteric ischemia is rare and the symptoms are vague, leading to high mortality caused by delayed diagnosis.
- There are 4 causes of acute mesenteric ischemia: arterial embolism, arterial thrombosis, mesenteric venous thrombosis, and nonocclusive mesenteric ischemia.
- History, physical examination, and laboratory findings lack the sensitivity and specificity to exclude acute mesenteric ischemia. Only computed tomography angiography can rapidly and accurately confirm the diagnosis.
- Survival is associated with rapid diagnosis and surgical treatment involving restoration of perfusion and assessment of the bowel.
- Advances in imaging, operative techniques, and critical care have led to a steady decline in overall mortality.

## INTRODUCTION

Acute mesenteric ischemia (AMI) continues to challenge even the most astute clinicians.[1] Its vague, nonspecific symptoms overlap with common illnesses, resulting in delayed diagnosis and historically dismal survival rates.[2–4] In addition, advanced age and comorbidities in patients with AMI mean that, despite timely identification, mortality exceeds 50% in recent series.[5–7] The aging of society portends an inevitable increase in the incidence of AMI; therefore, physicians must maintain a thorough understanding of this disease.[8] This article reviews the presentation, diagnosis, and treatment of the 4 most common causes of AMI: arterial embolism (AE), arterial thrombosis (AT), mesenteric venous thrombosis (MVT), and nonocclusive mesenteric ischemia (NOMI).

Disclosure: The authors have nothing to disclose.

[a] Division of Trauma and Critical Care, Medical College of Wisconsin, 9200 West Wisconsin Avenue, Milwaukee, WI 53226, USA; [b] Division of Digestive Diseases, Emory University, 615 Michael Street, Suite 201, Atlanta, GA 30322, USA; [c] Division of Pulmonary and Critical Care Medicine, The Medical College of Wisconsin, Suite E 5200, 9200 West Wisconsin Avenue, Milwaukee, WI 53226, USA

* Corresponding author.

*E-mail address:* tcarver@mcw.edu

Crit Care Clin 32 (2016) 155–171
http://dx.doi.org/10.1016/j.ccc.2015.11.001
critical care.theclinics.com

## EPIDEMIOLOGY AND COMORBIDITIES ASSOCIATED WITH ACUTE MESENTERIC ISCHEMIA

The rates of AMI range from 0.1 to 1 per 1000 hospital admissions, depending on the origin of the report.[8,9] AMI is a disease of the elderly with a median age of 74 years,[10] and is more common than appendicitis in patients greater than 75 years of age.[11] The frequency of each cause varies greatly across studies,[4–6,12,13] but AE is no longer the most common cause.[14] Rates of AT and AE seem to be almost equal using data provided in the comprehensive review by Schoots and colleagues[10] (**Table 1**). AMI affects slightly more women (51.4%), but the gender ratio differs depending on the cause.[10]

As expected given the age of the cohort, comorbidities associated with AMI are common. Dahlke and colleagues[6] reported that 27% of patients had peripheral arterial disease and 46% had coronary artery disease. Hypertension, hyperlipidemia, diabetes, and obesity are also typically present.[6,15,16] Beaulieu and colleagues[16] found a Charlson Comorbidity Index of 1.13 to 1.53 in 2000 patients with AMI, scores that are associated with a 25% 1-year mortality, further emphasizing the impact of disease burden on the AMI population.

## CLINICAL PRESENTATION OF ACUTE MESENTERIC ISCHEMIA

The typical presentation is an elderly person with multiple comorbidities, complaining of severe abdominal pain out of proportion to the examination. Although pain is the most consistent symptom, clinicians must appreciate that the presentation varies significantly depending on the cause of AMI (**Table 2**).[12] Vomiting, diarrhea, distention, and blood in the stool occur frequently but not universally.[17–19] Altered mental status is common, complicating the evaluation of patients with AMI.[17]

The progression of symptoms from superior mesenteric artery (SMA) occlusion is well described.[20] Small bowel ischemia causes crampy, periumbilical pain, but tenderness on examination is minimal until transmural ischemia develops, at which point peritoneal signs become evident. Intestinal necrosis eventually develops, leading to diffuse peritonitis, a rigid abdomen, and sepsis. Note that peritonitis on examination is reported in as few as 16% of patients with necrotic bowel.[12] Bowel sounds do not reliably indicate disorder and may be present until late in the course.[21] The diagnosis remains challenging, illustrated by AMI being clinically suspected in only 22% of patients who died of the disease.[19]

## LABORATORY TESTS IN ACUTE MESENTERIC ISCHEMIA

White blood cell count, lactate, D-dimer, and metabolic acidosis are classic serum markers for AMI.[19] Leukocytosis is one of the most common laboratory abnormalities in AMI, with

**Table 1**
**Summary of AMI by cause**

| Cause | Incidence (%) | Median Age (y) | Female/Male | Mortality (%) |
|---|---|---|---|---|
| AT | 34 (13–68) | 72 (59–78) | 1.46 | 70 (27–100) |
| AE | 34 (17–64) | 69 (60–75) | 1.23 | 66 (18–88) |
| Venous thrombosis | 13 (2–26) | 70 (43–74) | 0.78 | 44 (25–69) |
| NOMI | 19 (5–52) | 69 (57–76) | 1.17 | 70 (50–83) |

*Data from* Schoots IG, Koffeman GI, Legemate DA, et al. Systematic review of survival after acute mesenteric ischaemia according to disease aetiology. Br J Surg 2004;91:17–27.

**Table 2**
**Common presenting symptoms and risk factors for AMI**

| Cause | Symptoms | Presentation | Risk Factors | Ref |
|---|---|---|---|---|
| AE | Acute-onset abdominal pain<br>Nausea/vomiting<br>Diarrhea<br>Hematochezia | Pain out of proportion<br>Distention<br>Tachycardia<br>Hypotension<br>Peritonitis | Atrial fibrillation<br>History of MI, CHF<br>Recent cardiac or vascular surgery<br>Prior embolism in one-third | 2,12,17,21,33,41 |
| AT | Progressively worsening pain<br>Nausea/vomiting<br>Food fear<br>Postprandial pain<br>Weight loss | Pain out of proportion<br>Distention<br>Tachycardia<br>Hypotension<br>Peritonitis | CMI symptoms 20%–65%<br>History of CAD<br>PAD<br>Tobacco use | 2,12,13,17,20,21,33,41 |
| Venous thrombosis | Insidious onset<br>Vague abdominal pain Nausea/vomiting<br>May be asymptomatic | Vague tenderness<br>GI bleeding:<br>• Upper 10%<br>• Lower 16%<br>Peritonitis | Prior DVT or PE in 50%<br>Recent abdominal surgery<br>Hypercoagulable state<br>BCP | 3,18,35,36 |
| NOMI | Critically ill patient<br>Abdominal pain<br>Hypotension<br>Altered mental status<br>Diarrhea | Tenderness<br>Distention<br>Feeding intolerance | Recent cardiac surgery<br>ESRD<br>CHF<br>Digitalis<br>Vasopressors | 21,26,64 |

*Abbreviations:* BCP, birth control pills; CAD, coronary artery disease; CHF, congestive heart failure; CMI, chronic mesenteric ischemia; DVT, deep venous thrombosis; ESRD, end-stage renal disease; GI, gastrointestinal; MI, myocardial infarction; PAD, peripheral artery disease; PE, pulmonary embolism.

75% of patients having white blood cell counts exceeding 15,000/cells/mm$^3$.[17] However, even profound leukocytosis fails to differentiate AMI from other diagnoses.[22] Metabolic acidosis may not always be present; metabolic alkalosis may occur more frequently in early AMI because of vomiting.[23]

The failure of traditional laboratory tests has led researchers to identify biomarkers released from the mucosa during early ischemia.[22] Although D-lactate and alpha-glutathione S-transferase lack diagnostic accuracy, intestinal fatty acid binding protein (I-FABP) offers promise.[22] Thuijls and colleagues[24] found that urinary I-FABP outperformed the classic markers in distinguishing AMI from other causes of abdominal pain (**Table 3**). However, I-FABP has not been validated in larger studies, and, because common laboratory tests for AMI cannot exclude the diagnosis, clinical suspicion for AMI mandates evaluation through radiological studies or surgical exploration.[22]

## IMAGING STUDIES IN ACUTE MESENTERIC ISCHEMIA

Abdominal plain films are regularly obtained during the initial evaluation of patients with AMI. Thumb printing, pneumatosis, free air, and/or portal venous gas on radiograph are usually only present once bowel necrosis has occurred, and 25% of people with AMI have normal abdominal radiographs.[18,25] Therefore, the role of abdominal radiographs in the evaluation of AMI is limited to excluding other causes of pain.[2]

**Table 3**
**Serum markers in AMI**

| Laboratory Test | Sensitivity (%) | Specificity (%) |
|---|---|---|
| WBC[22] | 80 | 50 |
| Lactate[19] | 86 | 44 |
| D-dimer[19] | 96 | 40 |
| pH[22] | 38 | 84 |
| Urine I-FABP[24] | 90 | 89 |

*Abbreviations:* I-FABP, intestine-fatty acid binding protein; WBC, white blood cell count.
*Data from* Refs.[19,22,24]

The avoidance of contrast and radiation give both magnetic resonance angiography (MRA) and ultrasonography appealing benefits compared with computed tomography (CT) angiography.[2] MRA lacks the resolution of CT, overestimates stenosis, and takes longer to obtain, decreasing its usefulness in AMI.[2] Although ultrasonography accurately detects mesenteric occlusion, obtaining adequate images in AMI is difficult because of distended loops of bowel.[26] Given the time necessary to perform the study and the likelihood of failure, ultrasonography for diagnosis of AMI is not recommended.[25]

Mesenteric angiography was the gold-standard for diagnosing AMI for decades, but has been replaced by CT angiography because of its excellent imaging quality, widespread availability, and ability to identify other abdominal disorders.[20] CT also identifies mucosal ischemia and small perfusion defects that were previously missed with traditional angiography.[27] The clear superiority of CT compared with other modalities was shown in a recent meta-analysis, which reported a sensitivity and specificity of 94% and 95%, respectively.[19] Nonetheless, traditional angiography remains an important tool as catheter-directed therapies for AMI continue to evolve.[2]

## MESENTERIC ANATOMY AND PHYSIOLOGY

Although the foregut, midgut, and hindgut are supplied by their respective arteries, a robust system of collaterals provides redundancy against vascular compromise (**Table 4**).[20,28,29] The superior mesenteric vein (SMV) provides venous drainage of

**Table 4**
**Distribution of mesenteric arteries and collaterals**

| Artery | Distribution | Collaterals |
|---|---|---|
| CA | Foregut: distal esophagus, stomach, first/second portion of duodenum | CA to SMA:<br>Pancreaticoduodenal arteries<br>Arc of Bühler (rare) |
| SMA | Midgut: third/fourth portion of duodenum, jejunum, ileum, colon to splenic flexure | CA to SMA: as above<br>SMA to IMA:<br>Arc of Riolan<br>Marginal artery of Drummond |
| IMA | Hindgut: descending colon to distal sigmoid colon | SMA to IMA: as above<br>IMA to iliac arteries:<br>Hemorrhoidal arteries |

*Abbreviations:* CA, celiac artery; IMA, inferior mesenteric artery.
*Data from* Walker TG. Mesenteric vasculature and collateral pathways. Semin Intervent Radiol 2009;26:167–74.

the small bowel and proximal colon, whereas venous return from the descending colon occurs through the inferior mesenteric vein. In contrast with the arterial collaterals, venous collaterals exist between other mesenteric veins and the systemic circulation, but they cannot compensate for acute SMV or portal vein thrombosis.[20]

Thirty percent of the postprandial cardiac output flows through the celiac artery (CA) and SMA, with 70% of the blood shunted to the metabolically active mucosa.[18,30] Tight control of intestinal perfusion occurs through multiple local and extrinsic signals at the capillary level.[18] Arteriolar tension receptors in the mesenteric vasculature can detect decreases in blood pressure and local production of metabolic byproducts like ADP, $CO_2$, and $H^+$, both leading to vasodilation and improved oxygen delivery.[18,31] The mesenteric vasculature responds to a variety of hormones, discussed later, which all have profound effects on perfusion.[18] However, compensatory mechanisms cannot overcome every ischemic insult, and, when they fail, AMI develops.

## PATHOPHYSIOLOGY OF ACUTE MESENTERIC ISCHEMIA

Thromboembolic disease of the SMA accounts for 80% of AMI in some reports.[32,33] Almost all emboli originate from the heart, preferentially affecting the SMA because of its angle off the aorta.[2,20] Ottinger[4] divided the SMA into 4 regions (origin, main trunk and middle colic artery (MCA), distal to MCA, peripheral), with obstruction at each of these regions creating a typical pattern of bowel ischemia (**Fig. 1**).[34] In 50% of patients, the embolus lodges just distal to the middle colic branch, but 15% occlude the origin.[2] In contrast, AT almost universally occurs at the SMA origin, the site of atherosclerotic plaque.[2,20] AT is a gradual process, beginning with stenosis of the SMA before thrombosis occurs.[32] Collaterals develop in response to the progressively diminished flow and may perfuse the bowel after thrombosis until distal extension of the clot eliminates collateral inflow (**Fig. 2**).[20]

Although not associated with arterial obstruction, both MVT and NOMI can lead to bowel necrosis if untreated.[1,30] **Box 1** shows the most common conditions associated with MVT.[1,35] Patients with MVT develop ischemia once venous congestion inhibits arteriolar perfusion at the capillary bed.[36] Large vein thrombosis usually results from inflammation or vascular trauma, but hypercoagulable states are associated with clot formation within the venous arcades.[36] As noted by Harnik and Brandt,[36] intestinal infarction is more likely to occur in the hypercoagulable group because fewer collaterals exist at the periphery. NOMI occurs as the combination of low cardiac output and vasoconstriction leads to inadequate $O_2$ delivery.[18] Animal models of NOMI show microcirculatory abnormalities between adjacent villi, potentially explaining the patchy ischemic distribution noted macroscopically.[30]

Increased oxygen extraction initially maintains mucosal integrity, even with a 75% reduction in blood flow.[19,37] However, with prolonged ischemia the mucosal barrier breaks down, bacterial translocation occurs, polymorphonuclear leukocytes (PMNs) are activated, and inflammatory pathways involving nuclear factor-kappa beta, interleukin-6, and tumor necrosis factor alpha are upregulated, setting off a cascade of events that culminates in multiorgan system failure.[38] The production of reactive oxygen species (ROS) by PMNs results in additional tissue damage, especially following reperfusion (**Fig. 3**).[30,31,39]

Paradoxically, reperfusion can cause more tissue damage than prolonged periods of ischemia.[39] Oxygen delivery to ischemic areas increases production of ROS beyond the free radical scavenging capabilities of the local tissues.[30] Free radicals then

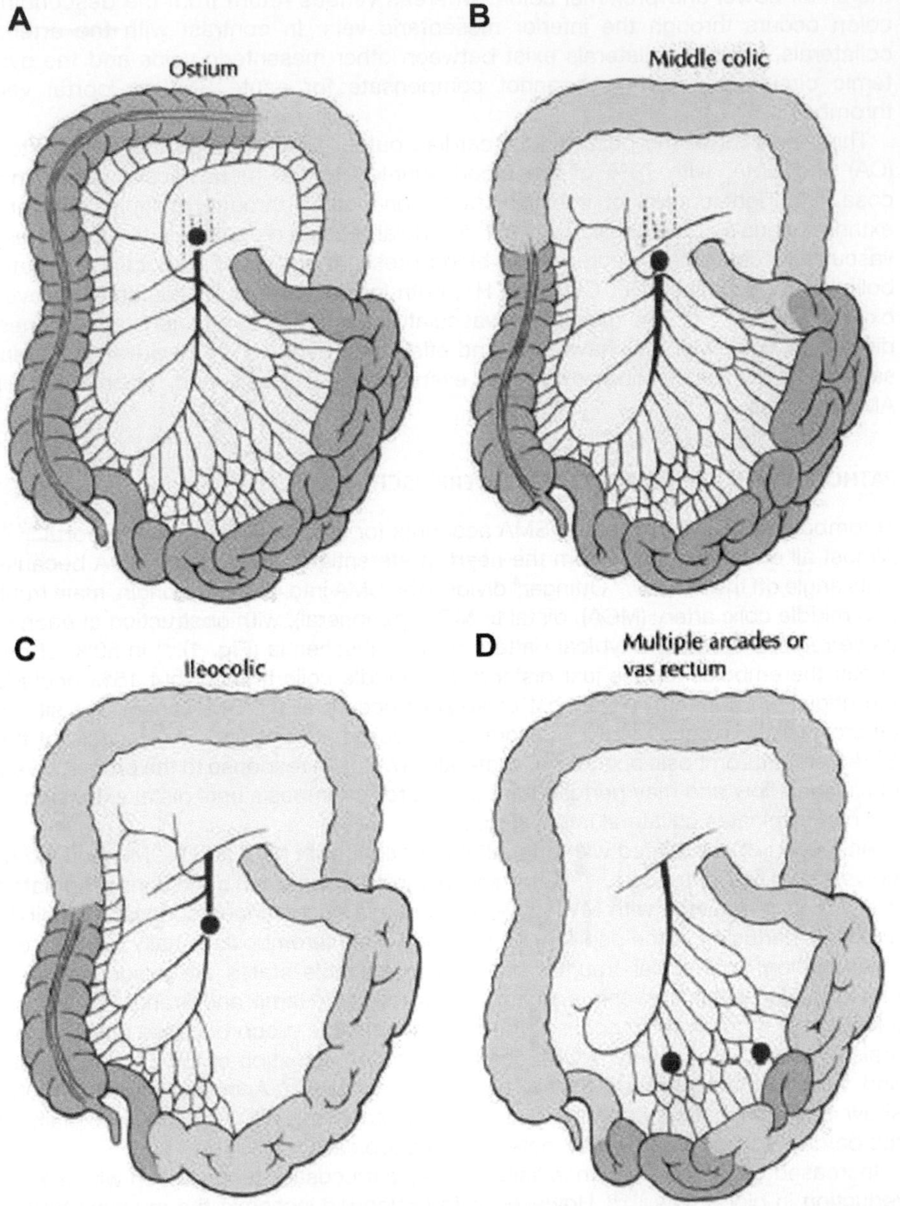


**Fig. 1.** Site of arterial occlusion and expected pattern of mesenteric ischemia. *A*. Occlusion at the SMA ostium leads to ischemia of the small bowel to the transverse colon. *B*. Occlusion distal to the MCA results in ischemia of the small bowel and the proximal ascending colon with sparing of the proximal small bowel. *C*. Occlusion in the distal ileocolic artery results in ischemia of the distal ileum and proximal ascending colon. *D*. Occlusion in distal branches results in focal intestinal ischemia. (*From* Donaldson MC. Mesenteric vascular disease. In: Creager MA, Barunwald E, eds. Atlas of vascular disease. 2nd edition. Philadelphia: Current Medicine Group; 2003. p. 117; with permission.)

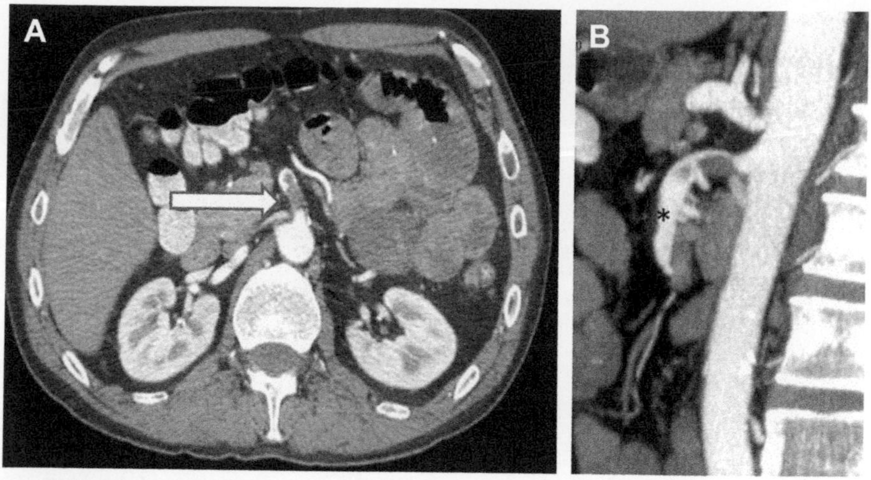


**Fig. 2.** (*A*) CT angiogram showing SMA thrombus (*arrow*). (*B*) Contrast is seen in distal SMA from collateral vessels (*asterisk*).

**Box 1**
**Causes of MVT**

*Hypercoagulable states*

- Antithrombin III deficiency
- Protein C/S deficiency
- Factor V Leiden
- Prothrombin 20210A gene
- Malignancy
- Polycythemia vera
- Oral contraceptives

*Direct injury or inflammation*

- Major abdominal surgery
- Blunt trauma
- Pancreatitis
- Inflammatory bowel disease
- Cholecystitis

*Venous stasis*

- Budd-Chiari
- Cirrhosis
- Postsplenectomy

*Data from* Morasch MD, Ebaugh JL, Chiou AC, et al. Mesenteric venous thrombosis: a changing clinical entity. J Vasc Surg 2001;34:680–4.

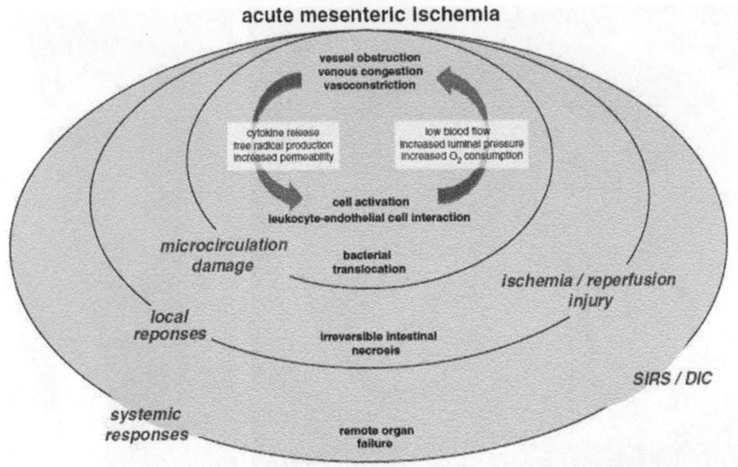


**Fig. 3.** Local and systemic response to AMI. DIC, disseminated intravascular coagulation; SIRS, systemic inflammatory response syndrome. (*From* Vollmar B, Menger MD. Intestinal ischemia/reperfusion: microcirculatory pathology and functional consequences. Langenbecks Arch Surg 2011;396(1):14; with permission.)

dissipate into surrounding areas, propagating a vicious inflammatory cycle that injures previously undamaged cells.[30] Furthermore, cytokines enter the systemic circulation, causing inflammatory injury to remote organs like the liver and lungs.[39]

## INITIAL TREATMENT OF PATIENTS WITH ACUTE MESENTERIC ISCHEMIA

Prompt diagnosis is one of the most important treatments for AMI. Once identified, aggressive volume resuscitation is initiated to correct hypovolemia. Broad-spectrum antibiotics with anaerobic coverage are administered, because of the likelihood of bacterial translocation.[37] Therapeutically dosed heparin minimizes clot propagation and decreases the risk of embolization in patients with atrial fibrillation.[2,21,40] Vasopressor agents (especially alpha-agonists) are avoided until volume replacement has occurred, because additional vasoconstriction can worsen ischemia.[2] Prompt surgical involvement is necessary, because consultation more than 24 hours after hospital presentation was associated with significantly increased mortality (36% vs 69%).[41] Time from surgical evaluation to operation of more than 6 hours also increases mortality (odds ratio, 4.7), further reinforcing the need for rapid treatment.[41]

## OPEN SURGICAL TREATMENT OF ACUTE MESENTERIC ISCHEMIA

Three principles guide the surgical management of thromboembolic AMI: SMA revascularization, assessment of intestinal viability, and resection of necrotic bowel. The patient's condition dictates the extent of the preoperative evaluation. Diffuse peritonitis or concern for necrotic bowel necessitates surgery without any additional evaluation.[27]

Assuming that the entire small bowel is not infarcted, the surgeon assesses for a pulse in the SMA. Revascularization, if necessary, is performed once the specific cause is established. Two recent articles detailed the surgical techniques used to treat AMI from arterial occlusion.[5,20] Following restoration of blood flow, the surgeon uses appearance of the tissue, presence of peristalsis, and pulsation at the periphery to determine intestinal viability, subjective findings that have a sensitivity of 82% and a specificity of 91%.[42] Injected fluorescein and detection of Doppler signals on the antimesenteric border may help identify perfused bowel, but studies regarding their utility are conflicting.[43,44]

Operative treatment of MVT or NOMI is reserved for patients with bowel necrosis, occurring in ~20% of patients with MVT.[21,45,46] Open SMV thrombectomy is complicated by frequent rethrombosis and does not improve survival.[47,48] Heparin plays a key role in MVT, because heparinization is associated with decreased rates of mortality, amount of resected bowel, and length of stay.[43] Although venous congestion causes a disconcerting appearance of the intestines, anticoagulation often results in macroscopic improvement within hours.[45]

Necrotic bowel is resected at the initial operation, but intestine of questionable viability should be left for reevaluation the next day.[20,27,47] In light of the frequent need for additional resection and the low risk of complications following damage control laparotomy,[49] temporary abdominal closure at the first procedure is recommended in all but the most straightforward situations.[1,21,29,33,43]

## ENDOVASCULAR TREATMENT OF ACUTE MESENTERIC ISCHEMIA

In 1977, Boley and colleagues[50] published one of the first reports of endovascular treatment in AMI. Refinements in techniques over the subsequent 40 years have led to the proliferation of endovascular procedures in patients with AMI.[51–53] A review of surgical treatment of AMI from 1999 to 2006 showed a 6-fold increase in endovascular therapies (primarily angioplasty with or without stenting) over the last 3 years of the report.[51] Two separate studies used the Nationwide Inpatient Sample (NIS) to evaluate the effect of endovascular treatment on AMI outcomes.[16,54] Despite advances in endovascular treatment, open surgery was used in 64.5% and 75.7% of patients. The endovascular cohort of those studies had improved survival and shorter length of stay, less need for total parenteral nutrition, and lower rates of renal and respiratory failure.[16,54]

The treatment of MVT with catheter-directed thrombolysis has mixed results in the literature. Although most patients respond to medical management alone, occasionally complications develop because of chronic venous thrombosis. The risk of these sequelae prompted some investigators to advocate for thrombolysis.[3,55] A randomized controlled trial comparing anticoagulation and thrombolysis with anticoagulation alone found that thrombolysis restored flow in 89% of patients.[3] Only 1 of 18 patients with thrombolysis required bowel resection versus 5 of 14 patients in the control group. In addition, 11% in the thrombolysis group versus 50% of the control group developed portal hypertension.[3] In contrast, Hollingshead and colleagues[55] showed complete lysis in only 15% of patients, and cavernous transformation in 85% of those without a complete response. Major complications related to thrombolysis occurred in 60%. In light of the differing findings, more studies are necessary to establish the efficacy of thrombolysis to treat MVT.

## NONSURGICAL TREATMENT OF ACUTE MESENTERIC ISCHEMIA

Although surgical therapy remains the mainstay of arterial AMI treatment, pharmaceutical therapies exist that can mitigate the effects of vasoconstriction and ischemia/reperfusion on patient outcome. Vasoconstriction associated with AMI prolongs ischemia even after blood flow is restored.[37,50] In addition to thromboembolic events, literature shows that vasoconstriction occurs in MVT, sepsis, and other shock states associated with NOMI.[40] The sympathetic nervous system is not the sole driver of splanchnic blood flow, and evidence confirms that the renin-angiotensin axis, vasopressin, and endothelin-1 all cause mesenteric vasoconstriction, even in the setting of alpha-blockade.[30,37,40,56] ACE inhibitors, glucagon, and endothelin-1 antagonists have shown benefit in animal models, but no human trials exist to support their use in AMI.[30]

Papaverine has been used to treat AMI-associated vasospasm since the 1970s, and it decreased NOMI mortality from 90% to 40% in one study.[50] As a phosphodiesterase inhibitor, papaverine increases cyclic AMP levels, resulting in nonselective vasodilation.[37] However, papaverine infusion into the SMA requires angiography, which may not be available in all institutions. In contrast, the vasodilator prostaglandin $E_1$ ($PGE_1$) provides an attractive alternative, because $PGE_1$ is administered intravenously. Mitsuyoshi and colleagues[56] used $PGE_1$ in 9 of 22 patients with AMI, noting a 78% survival rate compared with a 30% survival rate in the 13 controls. These encouraging initial results of $PGE_1$ in AMI must be studied further before recommending widespread use.

Altering the ischemia/reperfusion-induced injury is another target for therapy. Xanthine oxidase catalyzes the production of most free radicals, and animals treated with allopurinol have less epithelial damage following reperfusion.[37,40] Free radical scavengers like superoxide dismutase, nitroglycerine, *N*-acetyl cysteine, vitamin E, and glutamine have also shown benefit in animal models but are of limited clinical applicability, because most require pretreatment to be protective.[18,30,37,39,40]

Distant ischemic postconditioning decreases inflammatory markers in a variety of conditions associated with ischemia/reperfusion injury, including sepsis, myocardial infarction, and even traumatic brain injury.[57] Although not well understood, brief periods of induced ischemia following reperfusion decrease production of ROS.[58,59] In animals, ischemic postconditioning following mesenteric ischemia has shown decreased bacterial translocation, mucosal injury, and levels of inflammatory cytokines.[59]

## OUTCOME IN ACUTE MESENTERIC ISCHEMIA

Mortalities of up to 80% have been reported as recently as 1999[10] but vary considerably depending on the cause (see **Table 1**). Complications following treatment of AMI, such as respiratory failure, multiorgan system failure, sepsis, and short gut syndrome, affect 35% to 79% of patients,[6,13,19,29,33,60] and are associated with increased mortality.[6] Several other risk factors of mortality have been described, most notably age greater than 60 years, bowel resection, colon involvement, and duration of symptoms before treatment.[12,13,47,61,62] Beaulieu and colleagues[16] showed a 70% mortality if time to diagnosis was more than 24 hours versus a 14% mortality if less than 12 hours, confirming the importance of treatment before profound physiologic derangement occurs.

An NIS study showed that the in-hospital mortality of AMI decreased significantly after the year 2000 (49 vs 30%), a finding that was confirmed in Schoots and colleagues'[10] meta-analysis (**Fig. 4**).[10,54] Despite these improvements, AMI is associated with poor long-term survival.[13] Because recurrent arterial AMI is rare,[63] patients' comorbidities likely decrease long-term survival, as shown by the 20% and 70% 5-year survival in thrombotic and embolic AMI, respectively.[26] In the setting of significant comorbidities, physicians must consider the high morbidity and poor long-term survival before initiating aggressive treatment.

## PROGNOSTIC SCORING SYSTEMS IN ACUTE MESENTERIC ISCHEMIA

Using a logistic regression model, Haga and colleagues[8] developed a simplified scoring system to predict mortality (**Table 5**). Despite using only 3 variables, the model has a receiver operator curve (ROC) of 0.8, comparable with the ROC of the Acute Physiology and Chronic Health Evaluation 2 (APACHE 2) score, but is much easier to use.[8]

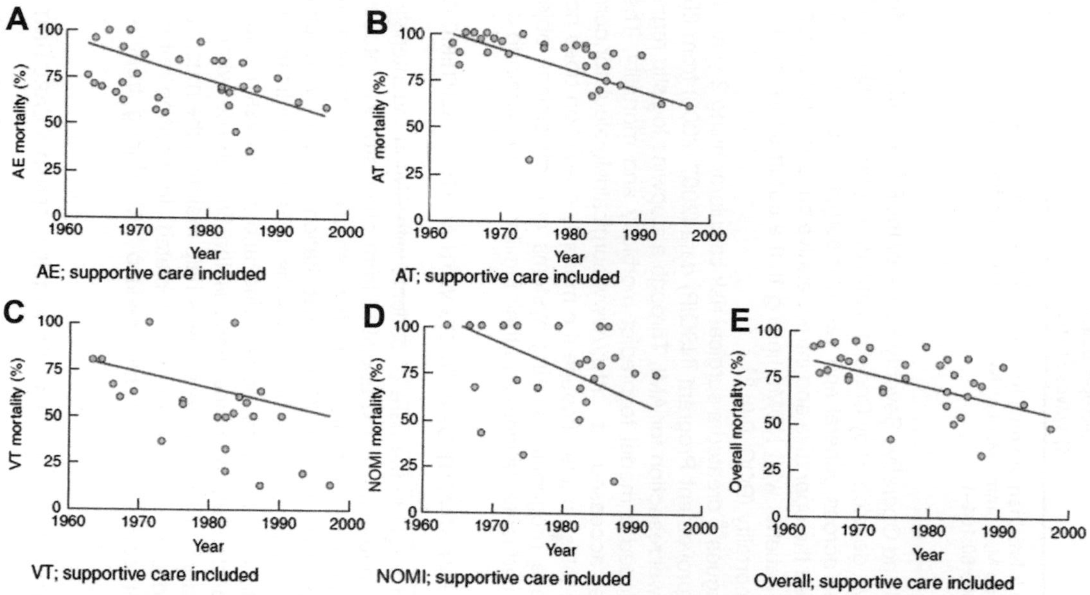


**Fig. 4.** Trends in AMI mortality by cause. (*A*) AE; (*B*) AT; (*C*) venous thrombosis (VT); (*D*) NOMI; (*E*) overall. (*From* Schoots IG, Koffeman GI, Legemate DA, et al. Systematic review of survival after acute mesenteric ischaemia according to disease aetiology. Br J Surg 2004;91(1):23; with permission.)

**Table 5**
**Simplified score predicting AMI mortality**

| Score | Age (y) | electrocardiogram | Shock Index |
|---|---|---|---|
| 1 | ≥70 | — | — |
| 2 | — | Atrial fibrillation rate 60–90/min | ≥0.7 |
| 4 | — | Other abnormal rhythm, >4 ectopic beats/min<br>Q waves/ST changes | — |

Mortality if total score is less than or equal to 2, 19%; 3 to 4, 37%; ≥5, 91%.

*Data from* Haga Y, Odo M, Homma M, et al. New prediction rule for mortality in acute mesenteric ischemia. Digestion 2009;80:104–11.

The Physiological and Operative Severity Score for the Enumeration of Mortality and Morbidity (POSSUM), developed by Copeland and colleagues in 1991, has been used to predict outcomes across general and vascular surgery procedures. Yukaya and colleagues[64] adapted the operative and intraoperative parameters to predict postoperative mortality in patients with NOMI, finding that a cutoff score of 76.1 best predicted in-hospital mortality (ROC, 0.9).[64]

Gupta and colleagues[65] created a surgical risk calculator using 2 years of National Surgical Quality Improvement Program (NSQIP) data (2007–2008) from 861 patients who underwent bowel resection for AMI. Through a stepwise logistic regression, the investigators developed a model to predict morbidity and mortality. The model is free and can be accessed at http://www.surgicalriskcalculator.com/ami-risk-calculator. This model is unique because the mortality prediction does not rely on a cutoff value.[65] These prognostic scoring systems give physicians objective data that can be used to educate patients and their families about expected outcomes.

## INTENSIVE CARE MANAGEMENT OF PATIENTS WITH ACUTE MESENTERIC ISCHEMIA

No large trials exist to guide the care of patients with AMI in the intensive care unit (ICU); therefore, management is extrapolated from other studies. Intubation, rather than noninvasive, positive pressure ventilation, should be performed in a patient with AMI with respiratory distress. Fluid resuscitation guided by dynamic markers rather than central venous pressure decreases the risk and complications associated with volume overload.[66] Because epinephrine and vasopressin cause profound splanchnic vasoconstriction, norepinephrine is the first choice when vasopressor agents are necessary.[67] Trophic enteral feeds help maintain the mucosal barrier but should be withheld until resuscitation is completed. In addition, intensivists must remain aware that some ICU patients develop AMI during treatment of other conditions.

## ACUTE MESENTERIC ISCHEMIA OCCURRING IN THE INTENSIVE CARE UNIT

Cardiac surgery is complicated by NOMI in 0.16% to 9% of patients, with several risk factors (**Box 2**).[68,69] Cardiopulmonary bypass results in hypoperfusion, generation of microthrombi, and reperfusion injury, all of which can lead to AMI.[69,70] Four findings are associated with AMI in patients after cardiac surgery: no bowel movement for 3 days after surgery, severe abdominal distention, radiography consistent with ileus, and increased lactate levels. The presence of any of these raises the concern for NOMI and appropriate imaging should be obtained.[71]

**Box 2**
**Risk factors for mesenteric ischemia after cardiac surgery**

- Age greater than 70 years
- Peripheral vascular disease
- Prolonged cross-clamp and bypass time
- Use of intra-aortic balloon pump
- Inotropic agents
- Postoperative blood transfusion greater than 2 units
- Postoperative renal failure
- Reexploration for bleeding

*Data from* Rodriguez R, Robich MP, Plate JF, et al. Gastrointestinal complications following cardiac surgery: a comprehensive review. J Card Surg 2010;25:188–97.

AMI in patients on dialysis has an incidence of 0.8% to 1.9% and is associated with both peritoneal dialysis and hemodialysis (HD).[72] Hypotension during HD in the ICU occurs in 43% of patients,[73] placing them at risk for developing AMI. Because the pain associated with dialysis-induced NOMI develops within 12 hours of HD, any patient with new or unexplained abdominal complaints after dialysis should be evaluated for AMI.[72]

## SUMMARY

The incidence of AMI will increase as the population ages, highlighting the importance of familiarity with this uncommon disease. Prompt treatment is associated with improved mortality, and CT angiography is the best test to diagnose AMI. Ongoing research and advances in surgical techniques, critical care, and pharmacologic therapy have led to an improvement in survival, but mortality will remain high until the diagnosis is routinely made before bowel necrosis has occurred.

## REFERENCES

1. Rhee RY, Gloviczki P, Mendonca CT, et al. Mesenteric venous thrombosis: still a lethal disease in the 1990s. J Vasc Surg 1994;20:688–97.
2. Wyers MC. Acute mesenteric ischemia: diagnostic approach and surgical treatment. Semin Vasc Surg 2010;23:9–20.
3. Di Minno MN, Milone F, Milone M, et al. Endovascular thrombolysis in acute mesenteric vein thrombosis: a 3-year follow-up with the rate of short and long-term sequaelae in 32 patients. Thromb Res 2010;126:295–8.
4. Ottinger LW. The surgical management of acute occlusion of the superior mesenteric artery. Ann Surg 1978;188:721–31.
5. Ryer EJ, Kalra M, Oderich GS, et al. Revascularization for acute mesenteric ischemia. J Vasc Surg 2012;55:1682–9.
6. Dahlke MH, Asshoff L, Popp FC, et al. Mesenteric ischemia–outcome after surgical therapy in 83 patients. Dig Surg 2008;25:213–9.
7. Leone M, Bechis C, Baumstarck K, et al. Outcome of acute mesenteric ischemia in the intensive care unit: a retrospective, multicenter study of 780 cases. Intensive Care Med 2015;41:667–76.

8. Haga Y, Odo M, Homma M, et al. New prediction rule for mortality in acute mesenteric ischemia. Digestion 2009;80:104–11.
9. Stoney R, Cunningham C. Acute mesenteric ischemia. Surgery 1993;114:489–90.
10. Schoots IG, Koffeman GI, Legemate DA, et al. Systematic review of survival after acute mesenteric ischaemia according to disease aetiology. Br J Surg 2004;91: 17–27.
11. Hansen KJ, Wilson DB, Craven TE, et al. Mesenteric artery disease in the elderly. J Vasc Surg 2004;40:45–52.
12. Acosta S, Block T, Bjornsson S, et al. Diagnostic pitfalls at admission in patients with acute superior mesenteric artery occlusion. J Emerg Med 2012; 42:635–41.
13. Kougias P, Lau D, El Sayed HF, et al. Determinants of mortality and treatment outcome following surgical interventions for acute mesenteric ischemia. J Vasc Surg 2007;46:467–74.
14. Meyers SI. Acute embolic and thrombotic mesenteric ischemia. In: Stanley J, Vieth F, Wakefield T, editors. Current Therapy in Vascular and Endovascular Surgery. 5th ed. Philadelphia: Elsevier; 2014. p. 718–20.
15. Marchena-Gomez J, Acosta-Merida MA, Hemmersbach-Miller M, et al. The age-adjusted Charlson Comorbidity Index as an outcome predictor of patients with acute mesenteric ischemia. Ann Vasc Surg 2009;23:458–64.
16. Beaulieu RJ, Arnaoutakis KD, Abularrage CJ, et al. Comparison of open and endovascular treatment of acute mesenteric ischemia. J Vasc Surg 2014;59: 159–64.
17. Burns BJ, Brandt LJ. Intestinal ischemia. Gastroenterol Clin North Am 2003;32: 1127–43.
18. Oldenburg WA, Lau LL, Rodenberg TJ, et al. Acute mesenteric ischemia: a clinical review. Arch Intern Med 2004;164:1054–62.
19. Cudnik MT, Darbha S, Jones J, et al. The diagnosis of acute mesenteric ischemia: a systematic review and meta-analysis. Acad Emerg Med 2013;20:1087–100.
20. Sise MJ. Acute mesenteric ischemia. Surg Clin North Am 2014;94:165–81.
21. Bobadilla JL. Mesenteric ischemia. Surg Clin North Am 2013;93:925–40, ix.
22. van den Heijkant TC, Aerts BA, Teijink JA, et al. Challenges in diagnosing mesenteric ischemia. World J Gastroenterol 2013;19:1338–41.
23. Acosta S, Nilsson T. Current status on plasma biomarkers for acute mesenteric ischemia. J Thromb Thrombolysis 2012;33:355–61.
24. Thuijls G, van Wijck K, Grootjans J, et al. Early diagnosis of intestinal ischemia using urinary and plasma fatty acid binding proteins. Ann Surg 2011;253:303–8.
25. McCarthy E, Little M, Briggs J, et al. Radiology and mesenteric ischaemia. Clin Radiol 2015;70:698–705.
26. Schwartz LB, Ng TT, McKinsey JF, et al. Diagnosis and surgical management of the visceral ischemic syndromes. In: Moore W, editor. Vascular and Endovascular Surgery. 8th ed. Philadelphia: Saunders; 2013. p. 423–36.
27. Renner P, Kienle K, Dahlke MH, et al. Intestinal ischemia: current treatment concepts. Langenbecks Arch Surg 2011;396:3–11.
28. Walker TG. Mesenteric vasculature and collateral pathways. Semin Intervent Radiol 2009;26:167–74.
29. Cho JS, Carr JA, Jacobsen G, et al. Long-term outcome after mesenteric artery reconstruction: a 37-year experience. J Vasc Surg 2002;35:453–60.
30. Kolkman JJ, Mensink PB. Non-occlusive mesenteric ischaemia: a common disorder in gastroenterology and intensive care. Best Pract Res Clin Gastroenterol 2003;17:457–73.

31. Vollmar B, Menger MD. Intestinal ischemia/reperfusion: microcirculatory pathology and functional consequences. Langenbecks Arch Surg 2011;396:13–29.
32. Acosta S. Mesenteric ischemia. Curr Opin Crit Care 2015;21:171–8.
33. Park WM, Gloviczki P, Cherry KJ Jr, et al. Contemporary management of acute mesenteric ischemia: factors associated with survival. J Vasc Surg 2002;35: 445–52.
34. Donaldson MC. Mesenteric vascular disease. In: Creager M, Braunwald E, editors. Atlas of Vascular Disease. 2nd ed. Philadelphia: Current Medicine Group; 2003. p. 111–27.
35. Morasch MD, Ebaugh JL, Chiou AC, et al. Mesenteric venous thrombosis: a changing clinical entity. J Vasc Surg 2001;34:680–4.
36. Harnik IG, Brandt LJ. Mesenteric venous thrombosis. Vasc Med 2010;15:407–18.
37. Kozuch PL, Brandt LJ. Review article: diagnosis and management of mesenteric ischaemia with an emphasis on pharmacotherapy. Aliment Pharmacol Ther 2005; 21:201–15.
38. Corcos O, Castier Y, Sibert A, et al. Effects of a multimodal management strategy for acute mesenteric ischemia on survival and intestinal failure. Clin Gastroenterol Hepatol 2013;11:158–65.e2.
39. Zabot GP, Carvalhal GF, Marroni NP, et al. Glutamine prevents oxidative stress in a model of mesenteric ischemia and reperfusion. World J Gastroenterol 2014;20: 11406–14.
40. Frishman WH, Novak S, Brandt LJ, et al. Pharmacologic management of mesenteric occlusive disease. Cardiol Rev 2008;16:59–68.
41. Eltarawy IG, Etman YM, Zenati M, et al. Acute mesenteric ischemia: the importance of early surgical consultation. Am Surg 2009;75:212–9.
42. Ballard JL, Stone WM, Hallett JW, et al. A critical analysis of adjuvant techniques used to assess bowel viability in acute mesenteric ischemia. Am Surg 1993;59: 309–11.
43. Yang S, Wu X, Li J. Transcatheter thrombolysis centered stepwise management strategy for acute superior mesenteric venous thrombosis. Int J Surg 2014;12: 442–51.
44. Urbanavicius L, Pattyn P, de Putte DV, et al. How to assess intestinal viability during surgery: a review of techniques. World J Gastrointest Surg 2011;3:59–69.
45. Brunaud L, Antunes L, Collinet-Adler S, et al. Acute mesenteric venous thrombosis: case for nonoperative management. J Vasc Surg 2001;34:673–9.
46. Acosta S, Ogren M, Sternby NH, et al. Fatal nonocclusive mesenteric ischaemia: population-based incidence and risk factors. J Intern Med 2006;259:305–13.
47. Endean ED, Barnes SL, Kwolek CJ, et al. Surgical management of thrombotic acute intestinal ischemia. Ann Surg 2001;233:801–8.
48. Bergqvist D, Svensson PJ. Treatment of mesenteric vein thrombosis. Semin Vasc Surg 2010;23:65–8.
49. Khan A, Hsee L, Mathur S, et al. Damage-control laparotomy in nontrauma patients: review of indications and outcomes. J Trauma Acute Care Surg 2013;75:365–8.
50. Boley SJ, Sprayregan S, Siegelman SS, et al. Initial results from an aggressive roentgenological and surgical approach to acute mesenteric ischemia. Surgery 1977;82:848–55.
51. Block TA, Acosta S, Bjorck M. Endovascular and open surgery for acute occlusion of the superior mesenteric artery. J Vasc Surg 2010;52:959–66.
52. Acosta S, Sonesson B, Resch T. Endovascular therapeutic approaches for acute superior mesenteric artery occlusion. Cardiovasc Intervent Radiol 2009;32: 896–905.

53. Arthurs ZM, Titus J, Bannazadeh M, et al. A comparison of endovascular revascularization with traditional therapy for the treatment of acute mesenteric ischemia. J Vasc Surg 2011;53:698–704 [discussion: 5].
54. Schermerhorn ML, Giles KA, Hamdan AD, et al. Mesenteric revascularization: management and outcomes in the United States, 1988-2006. J Vasc Surg 2009;50:341–8.e1.
55. Hollingshead M, Burke CT, Mauro MA, et al. Transcatheter thrombolytic therapy for acute mesenteric and portal vein thrombosis. J Vasc Interv Radiol 2005;16: 651–61.
56. Mitsuyoshi A, Obama K, Shinkura N, et al. Survival in nonocclusive mesenteric ischemia: early diagnosis by multidetector row computed tomography and early treatment with continuous intravenous high-dose prostaglandin E(1). Ann Surg 2007;246:229–35.
57. Joseph B, Pandit V, Zangbar B, et al. Secondary brain injury in trauma patients: the effects of remote ischemic conditioning. J Trauma Acute Care Surg 2015;78: 698–703 [discussion: 5].
58. Ferencz A, Takacs I, Horvath S, et al. Examination of protective effect of ischemic postconditioning after small bowel autotransplantation. Transplant Proc 2010;42: 2287–9.
59. Rosero O, Onody P, Kovacs T, et al. Impaired intestinal mucosal barrier upon ischemia-reperfusion: "patching holes in the shield with a simple surgical method". Biomed Res Int 2014;2014:210901.
60. Aliosmanoglu I, Gul M, Kapan M, et al. Risk factors effecting mortality in acute mesenteric ischemia and mortality rates: a single center experience. Int Surg 2013;98:76–81.
61. Yun WS, Lee KK, Cho J, et al. Treatment outcome in patients with acute superior mesenteric artery embolism. Ann Vasc Surg 2013;27:613–20.
62. Bjorck M, Acosta S, Lindberg F, et al. Revascularization of the superior mesenteric artery after acute thromboembolic occlusion. Br J Surg 2002;89:923–7.
63. Klempnauer J, Grothues F, Bektas H, et al. Results of portal thrombectomy and splanchnic thrombolysis for the surgical management of acute mesentericoportal thrombosis. Br J Surg 1997;84:129–32.
64. Yukaya T, Saeki H, Taketani K, et al. Clinical outcomes and prognostic factors after surgery for non-occlusive mesenteric ischemia: a multicenter study. J Gastrointest Surg 2014;18:1642–7.
65. Gupta PK, Natarajan B, Gupta H, et al. Morbidity and mortality after bowel resection for acute mesenteric ischemia. Surgery 2011;150:779–87.
66. Marik PE, Monnet X, Teboul JL. Hemodynamic parameters to guide fluid therapy. Ann Intensive Care 2011;1:1.
67. Hollenberg SM. Vasoactive drugs in circulatory shock. Am J Respir Crit Care Med 2011;183:847–55.
68. Groesdonk HV, Klingele M, Schlempp S, et al. Risk factors for nonocclusive mesenteric ischemia after elective cardiac surgery. J Thorac Cardiovasc Surg 2013;145:1603–10.
69. Rodriguez R, Robich MP, Plate JF, et al. Gastrointestinal complications following cardiac surgery: a comprehensive review. J Card Surg 2010;25:188–97.
70. Viana FF, Chen Y, Almeida AA, et al. Gastrointestinal complications after cardiac surgery: 10-year experience of a single Australian centre. ANZ J Surg 2013;83: 651–6.
71. Eris C, Yavuz S, Yalcinkaya S, et al. Acute mesenteric ischemia after cardiac surgery: an analysis of 52 patients. ScientificWorldJournal 2013;2013:631534.

72. Li SY, Chen YT, Chen TJ, et al. Mesenteric ischemia in patients with end-stage renal disease: a nationwide longitudinal study. Am J Nephrol 2012;35:491–7.
73. Akhoundi A, Singh B, Vela M, et al. Incidence of adverse events during continuous renal replacement therapy. Blood Purif 2015;39:333–9.

# Controversies in Critical Care Nutrition Support

Jayshil J. Patel, MD[a,*], Panna Codner, MD[b]

**KEYWORDS**

- Nutritional risk • Enteral nutrition • Parenteral nutrition • Trophic feeding
- Autophagy • Permissive underfeeding • Shock

**KEY POINTS**

- Nutritional risk is the risk of acquiring complications and other adverse outcomes that might have been prevented by timely and adequate nutrition support.
- In critically ill patients with an intact gut, early enteral nutrition (EN) is preferred to parenteral nutrition (PN).
- In low-risk patients with contraindications for EN, starting PN can be delayed for 7 to 10 days, but in high-risk patients with contraindications for EN, starting PN within 24 to 48 hours is reasonable.
- The exact timing for adding supplemental PN to hypocaloric EN remains controversial but, in high-risk patients, adding supplemental PN after day 7 is reasonable.
- Despite studies showing tolerability and lack of complications, further research is needed to evaluate dose and timing of EN in shock.

## INTRODUCTION

Critical illness predisposes individuals to highly variable metabolic and immune responses, leading to muscle mass loss, impaired healing, immobility, and susceptibility to infections and cognitive impairment.[1] Previously thought of as adjunctive therapy, nutrition support is a form of primary therapy in critically ill patients with both nutritional and non-nutritional benefits. Recommendations for nutrition in critically ill patients are supported by observational studies, small randomized controlled trials (RCTs), and mechanistic data.[2] Controversies such as the type, quantity, and timing

Disclosure: The authors have nothing to disclose.
[a] Division of Pulmonary & Critical Care Medicine, Department of Medicine, Medical College of Wisconsin, 9200 West Wisconsin Avenue, Milwaukee, WI 53226, USA; [b] Division of Trauma and Acute Care Surgery, Department of Surgery, Medical College of Wisconsin, 9200 West Wisconsin Avenue, Milwaukee, WI 53226, USA
* Corresponding author.
*E-mail address:* jpatel2@mcw.edu

Crit Care Clin 32 (2016) 173–189
http://dx.doi.org/10.1016/j.ccc.2015.11.002 criticalcare.theclinics.com
0749-0704/16/$ – see front matter 

of nutrition support and the role of nutrition during hemodynamic instability have limited the widespread application of nutrition support. This article reviews the physiologic basis for nutrition support and the concept of nutritional risk, and reviews various controversies in critical care nutrition support. This article does not discuss controversies in composition of nutrition support or nutrition support in specific disease subsets. The reader is referred to societal guidelines for a thorough review of these topics.[3,4]

## PHYSIOLOGIC BASIS FOR NUTRITION SUPPORT

In 1930, David Paton Cuthbertson described 3 successive phases of the metabolic response to critical illness. The first is an ebb phase, reducing basal metabolism. The second is a hypercatabolic flow phase, characterized by major protein catabolism, and leading to a reduced pool of muscle amino acids and glutamine. Third is an anabolic phase of muscle mass reconstruction, healing, and progression toward homeostasis.[1] However, at the onset of the anabolic phase, muscle atrophy may be severe and reduced muscle mass has been associated with poor intensive care unit (ICU) outcomes.[1,5]

The metabolic response to stress is complex and involves activation of neuroendocrine, inflammatory/immune, adipose tissue hormones, and gastrointestinal (GI) hormone components. The neuroendocrine component begins within seconds to minutes of the stress, activating the sympathetic nervous system and hypothalamic-pituitary axis. The inflammatory/immune components are activated within days, and lead to release of cytokines and inflammatory mediators such as tumor necrosis factor, interleukin-1, and interleukin-6. In addition to orchestrating the systemic inflammatory response syndrome (SIRS), these cytokines also induce weight loss, proteolysis, and lipolysis.[6] In addition, gene expression is altered in response to severe stress with increased expression of genes involved in the SIRS response and suppression of genes involved in adaptive immunity.[6] Adipokines (released from fat tissue) such as leptin, resistin, and adiponectin potentially contribute to the metabolic response to stress. In addition, levels of the GI tract hormone ghrelin are reduced and levels of cholecystokinin and peptide YY are increased.[6] Activation of these pathways ultimately leads to uncontrolled catabolism, insulin resistance, increased energy expenditure, and use of energy substrates (**Fig. 1**).

Uncontrolled catabolism leads to a cumulative calorie deficit. A negative cumulative energy balance has been associated with occurrence of acute respiratory distress syndrome, renal failure, need for surgery, and pressure sores.[7] The delivery of exogenous nutrients via the enteral or parenteral routes can provide sufficient calories; it can deliver micronutrients, and antioxidants for energy substrate repletion and maintenance of daily caloric balance. In addition, protein supplementation can restore protein stores and preserve lean body mass.[8]

However, it is enteral nutrition (EN), as opposed to parenteral nutrition (PN), that provides non-nutritional benefits (**Box 1**). Consider the consequences of not providing EN. In the absence of luminal nutrients, there is loss of structural and functional integrity.[8] Reduced gut contractility promotes bacterial overgrowth and increases bacterial virulence with contact-dependent programmed enterocyte apoptosis. Enterocyte death leads to structural defects, enhancing gut permeability for bacterial translocation and ultimately increasing the SIRS response.[8]

Providing EN maintains functional and structural integrity by stimulating intestinal contractility to sweep bacteria downstream and reduces bacterial overgrowth.

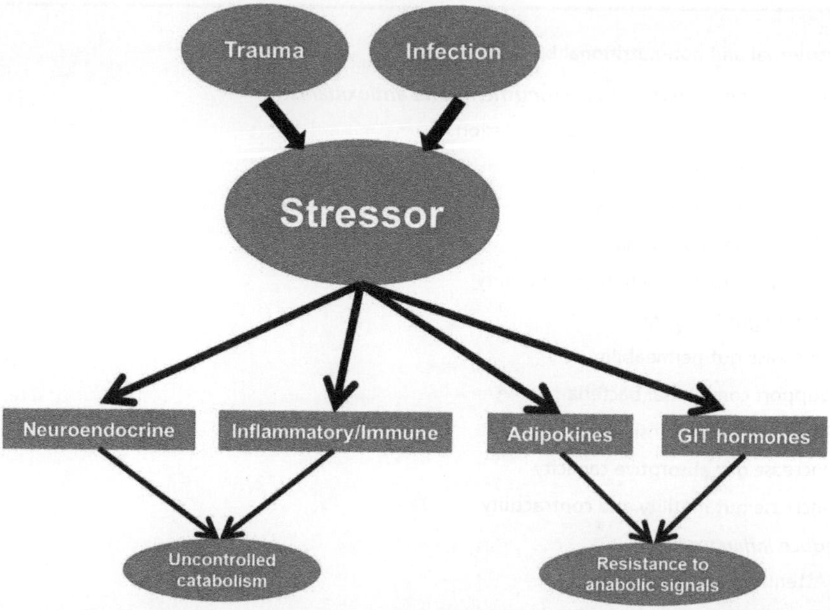


**Fig. 1.** The metabolic response to stress activates neuroendocrine hormones, inflammatory/immune hormones, adipokines, and GI tract (GIT) hormones. The consequence of the metabolic response is uncontrolled catabolism and resistance to anabolic signals. (*Adapted from* Preiser JC, Ichai C, Orban JC, et al. Metabolic response to the stress of critical illness. Br J Anaesth 2014;113(6):502.)

EN causes the release of trophic substances and stimulates gut blood flow to support gut-associated lymphoid tissue. EN stimulates immunity by releasing secretory immunoglobulin A. In addition, EN promotes commensal bacteria to provide direct protection by bacterial toxin degradation and increase butyrin production, the latter being known to reduce the inflammatory response.[8]

## NUTRITIONAL RISK

The metabolic stress response and preexisting nutritional state predispose critically ill patients to nutritional risk. Nutritional risk is the risk of acquiring complications and other forms of adverse outcomes that might have been prevented by timely and adequate nutrition support. Traditional nutrition assessment tools, such as albumin and prealbumin testing, are not validated in critical care for nutritional risk prediction.[4] In addition, classic variables such as body mass index (BMI), recent weight loss, and recent food intake only take into account preexisting nutritional state. A malnourished patient as identified by these classic variables should receive nutrition support. However, the aim for well-nourished ICU patients is to prevent malnourishment. Thus, for well-nourished patients, it is the metabolic stress that drives the indication for nutrition support.

Scoring systems incorporating variables associated with metabolic stress and preexisting nutritional status have been developed to determine nutritional risk (**Table 1**). The Nutritional Risk Screening (NRS) 2002 score is one such tool. Kondrup and colleagues[9] identified nutritional status and severity of illness variables from 128 randomized trials. To determine the total score, separate scores from nutritional status (0–3)

**Box 1**
**Nutritional and non-nutritional benefits of early EN**

*Provision of micronutrients/macronutrients and antioxidants*

- Decrease muscle and tissue glycosylation
- Increase mitochondrial function
- Increase protein synthesis
- Maintain lean body mass
- Enhance muscle function and mobility

*Maintain gut integrity*

- Decrease gut permeability
- Support commensal bacteria
- Promote insulin sensitivity
- Increase gut absorptive capacity
- Increase gut motility and contractility

*Reduce inflammation*

- Attenuate oxidative stress
- Reduce gut/lung axis of inflammation

*Preserve and enhance immunity*

- Maintain MALT tissue and increase secretory IgA
- Increase antiinflammatory Th-2 response
- Modulate adhesion molecules to decrease macrophage and neutrophil transendothelial migration

*Abbreviations:* IgA, immunoglobulin A; MALT, mucosal associated lymphoid tissue; Th-2, type 2 helper cells.

*Data from* McClave SA, Martindale RG, Rice TW, et al. Feeding the critically ill patient. Crit Care Med 2014;42(12):2600–10.

and severity of disease (0–3) categories are added together. If the age is greater than or equal to 70 years, an additional 1 point is added to the total score. If the age-corrected score is greater than or equal to 3, the patient is at nutritional risk and nutrition support commencement is recommended.[9]

Another tool is the Canadian Nutrition Risk in the Critically Ill (NUTRIC) score. Heyland and colleagues[10] identified 6 variables associated with nutritional risk: age, Acute Physiology and Chronic Health Evaluation II (APACHE II) and Sequential Organ Failure Assessment (SOFA) scores, number of comorbidities, pre-ICU length hospital length of stay (LOS), and interleukin-6 (IL-6) level. As opposed to the NRS 2002, the NUTRIC score does not take into account classic variables. NUTRIC only takes into account variables associated with a high degree of severity of disease.[11] The score has 6 elements, each assigning 0 to 2 points with higher scores (6–10, or 5–9 if IL-6 is not available) indicating higher risk for mortality (**Table 2**).

There are limitations with each nutritional risk assessment tool. For example, with the NRS 2002, any ICU patient with an APACHE II score greater than 10 is considered at nutritional risk independent of nutritional variables. The variable of ICU admission with APACHE score greater than 10 was drawn from an analysis of 5 RCTs with

**Table 1**
**Nutritional risk screening 2002**

| Impaired Nutritional Status | Severity of Disease |
|---|---|
| Normal nutritional status<br>Absent<br>Score 0 | Normal nutritional requirements<br>Absent<br>Score 0 |
| Weight loss >5% in 3 mo<br>Or<br>Food intake <50%–75% of normal requirement in preceding week<br>Mild<br>Score 1 | Hip Fracture<br>Chronic patients[a]<br>Mild<br>Score 1 |
| Weight loss >5% in 2 mo<br>Or<br>BMI 18.5–20.5 + impaired general condition<br>Or<br>Food intake 25%–50% of normal requirement in preceding week<br>Moderate<br>Score 2 | Major abdominal surgery, stroke, severe pneumonia, hematologic malignancy<br>Moderate<br>Score 2 |
| Weight loss >5% in 1 mo<br>Or<br>BMI <18.5 + impaired general condition<br>Or<br>Food intake 0%–25% of normal requirement in preceding week<br>Severe<br>Score 3 | Head injury<br>Bone marrow transplant<br>ICU patient (APACHE score >10)<br>Severe<br>Score 3 |

To calculate the total score: first, find the score (0–3) for impaired nutritional status and severity of disease; second, add the 2 scores for a total score; third, if age is greater than or equal to 70 years, add 1 point to the total score to correct for frailty of elderly; and fourth, if age-corrected total is greater than or equal to 3, start nutritional therapy.

*Abbreviation:* APACHE, acute physiology and chronic health evaluation.

[a] Cirrhosis, chronic obstructive pulmonary disease, chronic hemodialysis, diabetes, oncology.

*Data from* Kondrup J, Johansen N, Plum LM, et al. Incidence of nutritional risk and causes of inadequate nutritional care in hospitals. Clin Nutr 2002;21(6):461–8.

patients with trauma and burns with ICU LOS of at least 1 week.[11] However, there is no single variable that can predict ICU LOS across various ICU settings. A weakness of the NUTRIC score is its lack of a time-of-exposure criterion. Nutrition support would most benefit those patients who are exposed to a high degree of stress metabolism for a prolonged period of time.[11]

Optimizing nutrition support in patients with nutritional risk is important to mitigate complications and adverse outcomes. Observational studies have shown reduced complications in high-risk patients (as identified by NRS 2002 and NUTRIC scores) who received nutrition support, compared with those high-risk patients not receiving nutrition support.[12,13]

## LOCATION OF ENTERAL NUTRITION DELIVERY

EN can be delivered into the stomach, duodenum, or jejunum. Gastric feeding is typically delivered using a nasogastric or orogastric tube. In addition, percutaneous endoscopic gastrostomy (PEG) or surgical gastrostomy tubes can also be used to deliver

**Table 2**
**NUTRIC score variables**

| NUTRIC Score Variables | Range | Points |
|---|---|---|
| Age (y) | <50 | 0 |
| | 50 to <75 | 1 |
| | ≥75 | 2 |
| APACHE II score | <15 | 0 |
| | 15 to <20 | 1 |
| | ≥20 | 2 |
| SOFA score | <6 | 0 |
| | 6 to <10 | 1 |
| | ≥10 | 2 |
| Number of comorbidities | 0–1 | 0 |
| | 2+ | 1 |
| Days from hospital to ICU admit | 0 to <1 | 0 |
| | 1+ | 1 |
| Interleukin-6 (ng/mL) | 0 to <400 | 0 |
| | 400+ | 1 |

*Data from* Heyland DK, Dhaliwal R, Jiang X, et al. Identifying critically ill patients who benefit the most from nutrition therapy: the development and initial validation of a novel risk assessment tool. Crit Care 2011;15(6):R268.

EN to the stomach. Duodenal and jejunal EN delivery is considered postpyloric. The advantages and disadvantages of each delivery site are controversial. The primary theoretic disadvantage of nasogastric feeding is the increased risk of aspiration and subsequent pneumonia identified in studies in which tracheal secretions contained pepsin. Various strategies have been used to reduce aspiration risk. These strategies include postpyloric EN delivery, administration of motility agents, and elevation of the head of bed. The rationale for these strategies is based on the belief that gastroesophageal reflux increases the risk for nosocomial pneumonia. One study found no significant relationship between route of EN administration and aspiration risk.[14] Alternatively, in patients with severe cardiovascular failure, major burns, or more serious illness, a greater percentage of goal calories may be delivered postpylorically because large gastric residual volumes can result in feeding intolerance.[15,16] Practice patterns, contraindications, and ease of feeding tube placement continue to determine the location of feeding tubes in practice.

## EARLY VERSUS DELAYED ENTERAL NUTRITION

Timing is important to maximize EN provision advantages. Early EN is defined as feeding within 24 to 48 hours of initiating mechanical ventilation.[4] Early EN is thought to reduce inflammation and preserve enterocyte function, reducing infectious complications.[8] In addition, EN therapy serves as a vehicle to provide immune-modulating agents and acts as an effective means of stress ulcer prophylaxis.[4] In a large retrospective analysis of 4049 patients, Artinian and colleagues[17] reported that overall ICU and hospital mortalities were lower in critically ill medical patients who received early EN, defined as within 48 hours of mechanical ventilation (18.1% versus 21.4%, $P = .01$; and 28.7% vs 33.5%, $P = .001$, respectively). The lower mortalities were most evident in the sickest group, as defined by severity of illness score quartiles. Although Artinian and colleagues[17] reported an independently associated increased risk of ventilator-associated pneumonia in patients who received early EN, they advocated for the routine use of early EN in the sickest patients.

A meta-analysis of surgical patients who received early postoperative EN showed a reduction in infections (relative risk [RR], 0.72; 95% confidence interval [CI, 0.54–0.98; *P* = .03), reduced hospital LOS (mean, 0.84 days; range, 0.36–1.33 days; *P* = .01), and a trend toward reduced anastomotic dehiscence (RR, 0.53; 95% CI, 0.26–1.08; *P* = .08), compared with patients who received no postoperative nutritional support.[18]

A meta-analysis of 8 studies of early versus delayed EN studies among a heterogeneous group of critically ill patients reported improvement in mortality (RR, 0.52; 95% CI, 0.25–1.08; *P* = .08). Three studies reported a trend toward reduction in infectious complications (RR, 0.66; 95% CI, 0.36–1.22; *P* = .19). There were no differences in length of ICU stay.[3]

Future research to identify individuals at nutritional risk is needed to identify the patients who will derive the most benefit from early EN. Given the potentially large treatment effect with respect to mortality and reduction in infectious complications, major societal clinical practice guidelines continue to support early EN for critically ill patients.[3,4]

## AUTOPHAGY AND PERMISSIVE UNDERFEEDING

### *Autophagy*

Besides timing, EN quantity remains controversial. Optimal EN attenuates malnutrition and protein catabolism (which are associated with increased mortality), and achieving target goal calories improves patient outcomes.

Autophagy, first described in the 1970s, is a lysosomal process capable of removing damaged organelles, unfolded proteins, microorganisms, and excessive fat or carbohydrate stores. The process has been described as a system of quality control and may play a role in immunity, inflammation, and infection. Autophagy is regulated through stimulating factors such as starvation, oxidative stress, glucagon, and glutamine, and inhibitory conditions such as feeding, insulin secretion, hyperglycemia, and provision of excess nutrients.[19,20]

In critical illness, autophagy influences innate immune responses, generates inflammatory cytokines and interferon, stimulates the thymus gland, and promotes antigen presentation. However, the relationship between autophagy and the inflammatory immune arm is complex. Both play a role in inducing and suppressing the other, and both reduced and excessive autophagy are associated with cell death and adverse outcomes.[19] Identifying inhibition of autophagy during early nutritional therapy as the sole mechanism for adverse events is simplistic, and it is the interplay between autophagy and other physiologic systems in the body that determines overall outcome.[21]

The simple concept of stimulation of autophagy with starvation and inhibition with feeding is challenged by studies showing that nutrition inhibits autophagy in the liver (macroautophagy), releasing free fatty acids into the circulation and preventing intrahepatic fatty accumulation. Another example is found in protein synthesis, which is poor when derived from autophagic proteolysis.[19] Protein catabolism is directly correlated with disease severity and is not significantly influenced by starvation or feeding. On the contrary, whole-body protein synthesis is reduced during starvation.[22]

The relationship of autophagy to nutritional therapy was considered to be an explanation for the adverse effect of early nutritional therapy seen in a post-hoc analysis of the Early Parenteral Nutrition Completing Insufficient Enteral Nutrition in Adult ICU

Patients (EPaNIC) trial.[23] In critically ill patients receiving PN, less morbidity was observed with hypocaloric nutrition compared with standard nutrition.[24] By inhibiting autophagy, early full-dose EN therapy theoretically reduces mitochondrial function and tolerance to oxidative stress, and increases risk of multiple organ failure with cell death and increased mortality.[21] Briet and Jeejeebhoy[25] showed that protein refeeding, but not glucose refeeding, restores reduced mitochondrial function from malnutrition.

### *Permissive Underfeeding*

Permissive underfeeding is defined as restriction of nonprotein calories while supplying full protein requirements. With permissive underfeeding, the emphasis is to provide a sufficient level of protein intake during early critical illness to satisfy full protein requirements and meet metabolic demands.[26]

These aforementioned findings coincide with several past and present studies examining whether moderate caloric restriction with preservation of protein intake positively influences outcomes in critically ill patients. Studies examining the effect of EN quantity have yielded conflicting results.[27–31]

In a single-center RCT by Arabi and colleagues[32] a permissive underfeeding group was given 60% to 70% of the standard caloric requirement estimated using the Harris-Benedict equations and adjusting for stress factors, and the target feeding group received 90% to 100% of the standard caloric requirement. Protein dosed at 0.8 to 1.5 g/kg body weight was provided to both groups. To avoid protein malnutrition in the permissive underfeeding group, additional protein was added to maintain the full protein requirement without affecting the assigned caloric intake. Primary outcome of 28-day all-cause mortality was not statistically significant: 18.3% in the permissive underfeeding group compared with 23.3% in the target feeding group (RR, 0.79; 95% CI, 0.48–1.29; *P* = .34). Secondary outcome of in-hospital mortality was statistically significant: 30% in the permissive underfeeding group compared with 42.5% in the target group (RR, 0.71; 95% CI, 0.50–0.99; *P* = .04).[32]

More recently, Arabi and colleagues[33] again hypothesized that a permissive underfeeding strategy restricting nonprotein calories and preserving protein intake compared with a standard feeding strategy would decrease 90-day mortality among 894 randomized critically ill patients. The permissive underfeeding group received 40% to 60% of caloric requirements and the standard feeding group received 70% to 100% of caloric requirements. Protein requirements were calculated between 1.2 to 1.5 g/kg body weight per day. To ensure similarity of enteral protein and volume delivery between the two groups, the permissive underfeeding group received additional protein and normal saline or water. The standard feeding group required nonenteral caloric supplementation to achieve 70% target. The primary end point of 90-day mortality was not statistically significant: 27.2% in the permissive underfeeding group and 28.9% in the standard feeding group (RR, 0.94; 95% CI, 0.76–1.16; *P* = .58). Secondary end points including ventilator-free days, ICU-free days, and incidence of hypoglycemia did not differ significantly between the two groups. Clinical indices of protein status and nitrogen balance, based on prealbumin level, transferrin level, and urinary nitrogen excretion, were similar between the two groups. The investigators concluded that their results did not support the premise that higher caloric intake attenuated protein catabolism in critically ill patients.[33]

Trophic (or trickle) EN is an example of permissive underfeeding. Trophic EN has been studied in specific critical illness patient subsets. In patients with acute lung injury, 2 RCTs showed that trophic EN within 48 hours led to similar outcomes compared with patients receiving standard enteral feeding.[34,35] Trophic feeding does not provide adequate nutritional support over extended periods of time. The 2013 Canadian Critical Care Nutrition Guidelines report insufficient data to recommend hypocaloric EN in critically ill patients, whereas the 2009 Society of Critical Care Medicine (SCCM) and American Society of Parenteral and Enteral Nutrition Guidelines (ASPEN) recommend permissive underfeeding in critically ill obese patients.[3,4]

## PARENTERAL NUTRITION

PN is the delivery of calories, amino acids, electrolytes, vitamins, minerals, trace elements, and fluid via an intravenous route. Although EN is always preferable when nutritional therapy is provided, there is a role for PN in critically ill patients. Patient selection is important for optimizing the use of PN. For instance, PN may be reasonable in high-risk critically ill patients with an unreliable GI tract. A clear advantage to PN is that full nutritional requirements may be achieved within 12 to 24 hours.

### *Enteral Versus Parenteral Nutrition*

The most consistent outcome in studies of EN versus PN is reduction in infectious complications with EN.[36] Six meta-analyses comparing EN versus PN have shown significant reductions in infectious complications.[4] One meta-analysis by Simpson and Doig[37] showed lower mortality with EN (RR, 0.51; 95% CI, 0.27–0.97; $P$ = .04) despite a higher incidence of infectious complications (RR, 1.66; 95% CI, 1.09–2.51; $P$ = .02). More recently in the CALORIES trial, Harvey and colleagues[38] conducted a pragmatic multicenter RCT, randomizing 2400 patients to early EN or early PN. No significant differences were found in the primary outcome of 30-day mortality or secondary outcome of infectious complications. Less than 10% of patients in each group were malnourished, perhaps suggesting that these patients did not need either form of early nutrition support. Thus, in most critically ill patients with an intact gut, major societal guidelines recommend starting EN rather than PN (**Table 3**).[3,4,39] In nonmalnourished patients with contraindications for EN and/or oral intake, it is reasonable to initiate PN after 7 to 10 days (sometimes as late as 10–14 days).[4] In those at nutritional risk, starting early PN is reasonable, particularly if EN is not possible or contraindicated.

### *Supplemental Parenteral Nutrition*

Supplemental PN refers to the addition of PN to patients receiving insufficient or hypocaloric EN. Earlier studies of supplemental PN resulted in no difference in morbidity or mortality, ICU LOS, duration of mechanical ventilation, or incidence of respiratory infection.[40] One study showed an increase in mortality in patients who received supplemental PN, which was thought to be caused by a depression in T-cell helper-suppressor levels.[41]

More recently, 3 large RCTs showed conflicting results after adding supplemental PN to hypocaloric EN.[42–44] Two trials suggested that adding PN to hypocaloric EN derived no benefit compared with hypocaloric EN alone.[43,44] In the EPaNIC trial, Casaer and colleagues[42] compared early (within 48 hours after ICU admission) with late (8 days after ICU admission) PN. The late group experienced higher rates of being discharged alive from the ICU and from the hospital (hazard ratio [HR], 1.06; 95% CI, 1.00–1.13; $P$ = .04), fewer ICU infections (22.8% vs 26.2%; $P$ = .008), a 9.7% relative reduction in patients requiring more than 2 days of mechanical ventilation ($P$ = .006), and a median 3 fewer days of renal replacement therapy ($P$ = .008). After 14 days, patients on standard therapy (intravenous dextrose solution) without oral intake had

**Table 3**
**Recommendations for EN versus PN from major nutrition support guidelines**

| Guideline | Year | Recommendation for EN vs PN | Evidence |
|---|---|---|---|
| Canadian Critical Care Practice Guidelines | 2013 | When considering nutrition support for critically ill patients, the use of EN rather than PN is strongly recommended | Based on 1 level 1 and 13 level 2 studies |
| SCCM and ASPEN Guidelines | 2009 | EN is the preferred route of feeding rather than PN for critically ill patients who require nutrition support | Based on most level 1 and 2 studies |
| ESPEN guidelines | 2006 | All patients who are not expected to be on a full oral diet within 3 d should receive EN. Although there are no data showing improvement in relevant outcome parameters using early EN, the expert committee recommends hemodynamically stable critically ill patients who have a functioning GI tract should be fed early with appropriate amounts of EN | Based on level 1 studies |

*Abbreviation:* ESPEN, European Society of Enteral and Parenteral Nutrition.

increased mortality.[42] In the EPaNIC study, it is likely that adverse outcomes were caused by an effect of PN and not EN, because both groups were receiving an equal volume of EN delivery before initiating PN.[2]

In contrast, a small amount of EN during PN may attenuate gut atrophy and limit bacterial translocation.[45] PN in this setting can be tapered when the patient is able to tolerate more than 80% of protein and calories via the GI tract.

Overall, if a patient is at nutritional risk while receiving hypocaloric EN, adding supplemental PN at some point within the first week may be reasonable, the exact timing for which is unclear.

## NUTRITION SUPPORT IN SHOCK

For EN to be safely delivered and used there must be sufficient blood flow to the gastrointestinal tract. Critically ill patients are commonly hemodynamically unstable and requiring vasoactive support, putting them at risk for gastrointestinal hypoperfusion, EN intolerance, and nonocclusive mesenteric ischemia. Current critical care nutrition support guidelines provide none to weakly supported recommendations for early EN in critically ill patients with hemodynamic instability (**Table 4**).[46]

Current recommendations to withhold EN in patients with shock are based on 2 observations, both of which may increase risk of intestinal and vital organ ischemia reperfusion injury in hypotensive patients.

First, blood flow to the small bowel is such that the artery and vein of the villus run parallel, but their blood flows are in opposite directions (**Fig. 2**).[47] This anatomic arrangement allows countercurrent exchange of oxygen from the artery to the vein along the course within the villus. The result is a descending gradient of tissue partial pressure of oxygen ($Po_2$) from the base of the villus to its tip. Reduced blood flow

**Table 4**
**Recommendations for early EN from available nutrition support guidelines**

| Guideline | Year | Recommendations for EN in Shock | Limitations |
|---|---|---|---|
| Canadian Critical Care Practice Guidelines Committee | 2013 | The committee noted the results of a large observational study of 1174 critically ill patients on vasopressors and noted that those receiving early EN had decreased hospital mortality and that the benefit of early EN was more evident in those on multiple vasopressors, and the prerequisite that patients were adequately resuscitated (evidence level 16, 2 studies) | Selection bias in the stated observational study in which patients with poor ICU course received later EN |
| SCCM and ASPEN | 2009 | In the setting of hemodynamic compromise, EN should be withheld until the patient is fully resuscitated and/or stable, and EN may be provided with caution to patients either into the stomach or small bowel on stable low doses of vasopressor agents (grade E recommendation) | Lowest level of recommendation. There is no definition of low-dose vasopressor |
| ANZICS Clinical Trials Group Nutrition Guidelines | 2008 | No recommendations | NA |
| European Society for Clinical Nutrition and Metabolism | 2006 | Critically ill patients who were hemodynamically stable should be fed early (<24 h) (level C evidence) | Uncertain about hemodynamically unstable patients |

*Abbreviations:* ANZICS, Australian and New Zealand Intensive Care Society; NA, not-applicable.
*Adapted from* Yang S, Wu X, Yu W, et al. Early enteral nutrition in critically ill patients with hemodynamic instability: an evidence-based review and practical advice. Nutr Clin Pract 2014;29(1):90–6.

results in a lower $P_{O_2}$, leaving the tip of the villus susceptible to hypoxia. The small intestine is at a higher risk for ischemia than the colon because of this countercurrent exchange mechanism. Reduction of blood flow by greater than 50% is required before gut ischemia ensures.[47] The period of reperfusion may be a bigger factor in the injury to the gut than the initial period of ischemia.[48]

The second observation that gives rise to a theoretic objection to EN in hypotensive patients on vasopressors is that feeding may lead to a steal phenomenon by splanchnic circulation without an increase in total blood flow.[47,48]

Injury to villi tips may alter small bowel function in the absence of frank ischemia or necrosis. Because small bowel absorption involves villi tips, malabsorption occurs early and the osmotic effect of luminal formula leads to fluid shifts and diarrhea.

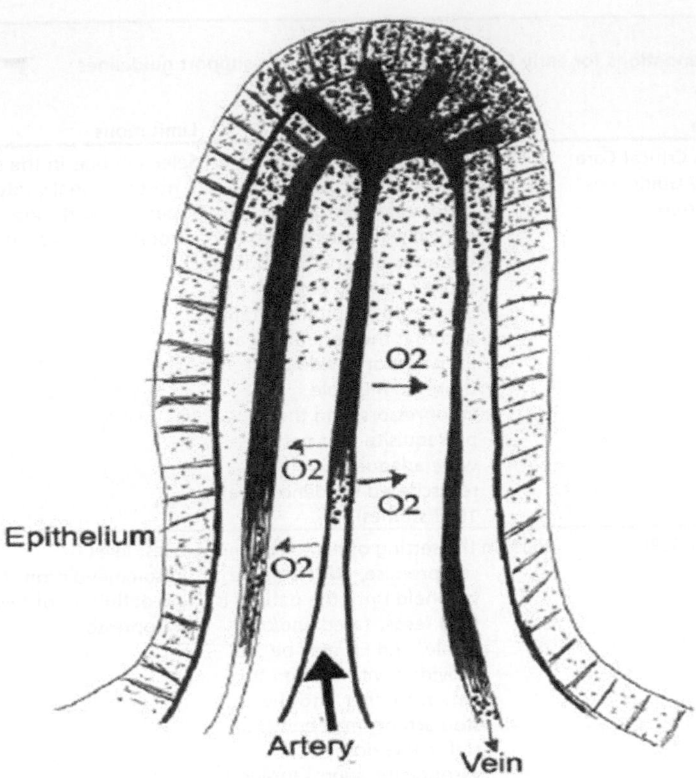


**Fig. 2.** Countercurrent exchange of oxygen in the intestinal villus. Oxygen diffuses from the artery to the villous veins throughout their course to the tip of the villus. This diffusion results in a descending partial pressure of oxygen ($Po_2$) gradient from the base to the villus to the tip. (*From* Takala J. Determinants of splanchnic blood flow. Br J Anaesth. 1997;77: 50–8; with permission.)

Subclinical ischemia may lead to reduced gut motility with consequential bacterial overgrowth, fermentation of formula, and gut distention. Bowel wall stretch promotes capillary sludging and decreased mucosal perfusion.[48] Gut integrity and barrier functions are jeopardized with promotion of bacterial translocation, endotoxemia, and accentuated inflammatory response.[8,49]

Animal studies show conflicting results as to whether EN in shock precipitates ischemic bowel. Rats provided luminal nutrients during hypotension showed increased jejunal hypoxia and mucosal permeability as well as decreased glucose absorption and metabolism. Clamping of the superior mesenteric artery established intestinal ischemia before institution of enteral nutrients.[50] Physiology in this model is different from feeding a patient with risk factors for, but not established, intestinal ischemia (because gastrointestinal ischemia occurs when blood flow is <50% the basal value). On the contrary, EN provided to dogs with endotoxin-mediated shock caused increased intestinal microcirculatory perfusion and increased blood flow to the portal vein within minutes of infusion.[51] Pretreatment with EN before ischemia may serve to reduce the degree of injury during hemodynamic instability. In dogs receiving 5 days of pretreatment with an elemental diet, subsequent hemorrhagic ischemia for 18 hours led to increased tolerance to ischemia and less mucosal injury compared with dogs given intact dog food.[52]

Human studies of cardiogenic shock have shown tolerance to EN.[53,54] Revelly and colleagues[53] evaluated the hemodynamic and metabolic adaptations to EN. Nine cardiothoracic surgery patients requiring hemodynamic support received isoenergetic postpyloric EN. EN increased cardiac index, splanchnic blood flow, and metabolic responses, showing that nutrients were used.[53] Berger and Chiolero[54] showed tolerance of greater than 1200 kcal/d EN in 70 post–cardiac surgery patients with circulatory failure requiring vasoactive support.

These studies provide observations in cardiogenic shock in which a reduction in splanchnic blood flow occurs in proportion to a reduction in cardiac output, putting the patient at risk for splanchnic ischemia. In septic conditions, the impact of blood flow reduction is unpredictable.[54] The addition of norepinephrine could lead to hepatosplanchnic vasoconstriction, placing the small bowel at risk for ischemia, but this mechanism may be offset by norepinephrine also increasing venous return by constriction of venous capacitance beds, thus increasing cardiac output.[55]

Data for EN in septic shock in humans are limited to retrospective and observational studies. Rai and colleagues[56] retrospectively studied 43 patients with sepsis (33 with shock) to determine the adequacy of EN in this population. EN was initiated at a mean of 1.3 days to 33 patients in shock with no differences in ICU or hospital mortality. The 33 patients with shock did have a larger mean residual volume, but this did not affect the success of feeding and complications were not reported.[56] Khalid and colleagues[57] showed improved ICU and hospital survival in the sickest of medical ICU patients (ie, those on multiple vasopressors) who had early EN compared with those with late EN. In a secondary analysis of the Intensive Insulin Therapy and Pentastarch Resuscitation in Severe Sepsis trial, 353 patients with severe sepsis or septic shock were evaluated to analyze the effect of 3 nutritional strategies.[58] Those receiving EN alone had improved 90-day mortality.[58]

Apart from the timing of EN, quantity of EN may be important. Rokyta and colleagues[59] showed that the initiation of low-dose postpyloric EN in ICU patients with severe sepsis led to the parallel increase in systemic and hepatosplanchnic blood flow, and that hepatosplanchnic energy metabolic, oxygen kinetics, and gastric mucosal energy did not deteriorate during EN. In a small retrospective study, Patel and colleagues[60] observed that less than 600 kcal/d in septic shock was associated with improved outcome of ICU LOS with no increased risk of complications secondary to EN, compared with no EN.

The gravest consequence of EN during shock is nonocclusive bowel necrosis (NOBN). NOBN has been mostly reported in critically ill patients receiving jejunal feeding.[46] Presumably, under conditions of bowel hypoperfusion or depressed peristalsis, the stomach could act as a buffering chamber, whereas jejunal retention worsens intraluminal tension and aggravate bowel ischemia. NOBN is rare, with a reported incidence of 0.29% to 1.14%, and the degree of risk for NOBN is difficult to determine based solely on vasoactive dose.[46]

Overall, trophic EN during shock may serve to maintain gut barrier and immune functions, mitigating the consequences of enhanced gut permeability and oxidative stress. Small-scale observations and descriptive and retrospective cohorts suggest tolerability and improvement in splanchnic perfusion and oxygenation in hemodynamically unstable patients. However, there are no large RCTs to answer questions of timing, dose, and route for EN delivery in shock. Furthermore, not all forms of shock are equal. Particularly, redistribution of blood flow is unpredictable in sepsis and higher quality data from studies investigating EN in different forms of shock are needed before further recommendations can be made.[54] Consensus statements maintain that volume resuscitation should take priority, with EN started at a trophic rate when the patient is on a stable or declining vasopressor dose.[3,4]

## SUMMARY

Critical illness is associated with significant metabolic stress. Consequences of metabolic stress include infectious complications, organ failure, and increased hospitalization and mortality. Nutrition support should be considered a form of therapy to reduce the consequences of metabolic stress. EN, as opposed to PN, should be started within 24 to 48 hours of ICU admission. In addition, nutritional risk should be determined to optimize nutritional support (eg, supplemental PN) in at-risk patients. There is no standardization of nutritional therapy in critically ill patients, possibly because of differences in patient population, disease subsets, local culture and practice, and institutional barriers. Future studies evaluating nutrition support timing, quantity, and composition should take into account these differences to better define which critically ill patients derive the most benefit from nutritional support.

## REFERENCES

1. Massanet PL, Petit L, Louart B, et al. Nutrition rehabilitation in the intensive care unit. JPEN J Parenter Enteral Nutr 2015;39(4):391–400.
2. McClave SA, Martindale RG, Rice TW, et al. Feeding the critically ill patient. Crit Care Med 2014;42(12):2600–10.
3. Dhaliwal R, Cahill N, Lemieux M, et al. The Canadian critical care nutrition guidelines in 2013: an update on current recommendations and implementation strategies. Nutr Clin Pract 2014;29(1):29–43.
4. McClave SA, Martindale RG, Vanek VW, et al. Guidelines for the provision and assessment of nutrition support therapy in the adult critically ill patient: Society of Critical Care Medicine (SCCM) and American Society for Parenteral and Enteral Nutrition (A.S.P.E.N.). JPEN J Parenter Enteral Nutr 2009;33(3):277–316.
5. Moisey LL, Mourtzakis M, Cotton BA, et al. Skeletal muscle predicts ventilator-free days, ICU-free days, and mortality in elderly ICU patients. Crit Care 2013;17(5):R206.
6. Preiser JC, Ichai C, Orban JC, et al. Metabolic response to the stress of critical illness. Br J Anaesth 2014;113(6):945–54.
7. Dvir D, Cohen J, Singer P. Computerized energy balance and complications in critically ill patients: an observational study. Clin Nutr 2006;25(1):37–44.
8. McClave SA, Heyland DK. The physiologic response and associated clinical benefits from provision of early enteral nutrition. Nutr Clin Pract 2009;24(3):305–15.
9. Kondrup J, Johansen N, Plum LM, et al. Incidence of nutritional risk and causes of inadequate nutritional care in hospitals. Clin Nutr 2002;21(6):461–8.
10. Heyland DK, Dhaliwal R, Jiang X, et al. Identifying critically ill patients who benefit the most from nutrition therapy: the development and initial validation of a novel risk assessment tool. Crit Care 2011;15(6):R268.
11. Kondrup J. Nutritional-risk scoring systems in the intensive care unit. Curr Opin Clin Nutr Metab Care 2014;17(2):177–82.
12. Heyland DK, Dhaliwal R, Wang M, et al. The prevalence of iatrogenic underfeeding in the nutritionally 'at-risk' critically ill patient: results of an international, multicenter, prospective study. Clin Nutr 2015;34(4):659–66.

13. Jie B, Jiang ZM, Nolan MT, et al. Impact of nutritional support on clinical outcome in patients at nutritional risk: a multicenter, prospective cohort study in Baltimore and Beijing teaching hospitals. Nutrition 2010;26(11–12):1088–93.
14. Metheny NA, Stewart BJ, McClave SA. Relationship between feeding tube site and respiratory outcomes. JPEN J Parenter Enteral Nutr 2011;35(3):346–55.
15. Berger MM, Revelly JP, Cayeux MC, et al. Enteral nutrition in critically ill patients with severe hemodynamic failure after cardiopulmonary bypass. Clin Nutr 2005; 24(1):124–32.
16. Sefton EJ, Boulton-Jones JR, Anderton D, et al. Enteral feeding in patients with major burn injury: the use of nasojejunal feeding after the failure of nasogastric feeding. Burns 2002;28(4):386–90.
17. Artinian V, Krayem H, DiGiovine B. Effects of early enteral feeding on the outcome of critically ill mechanically ventilated medical patients. Chest 2006;129(4):960–7.
18. Lewis SJ, Egger M, Sylvester PA, et al. Early enteral feeding versus "nil by mouth" after gastrointestinal surgery: systematic review and meta-analysis of controlled trials. BMJ 2001;323(7316):773–6.
19. Cuervo AM, Macian F. Autophagy, nutrition and immunology. Mol Aspects Med 2012;33(1):2–13.
20. Levine B, Mizushima N, Virgin HW. Autophagy in immunity and inflammation. Nature 2011;469(7330):323–35.
21. McClave SA, Weijs PJ. Preservation of autophagy should not direct nutritional therapy. Curr Opin Clin Nutr Metab Care 2015;18(2):155–61.
22. Berg A, Rooyackers O, Bellander BM, et al. Whole body protein kinetics during hypocaloric and normocaloric feeding in critically ill patients. Crit Care 2013; 17(4):R158.
23. Casaer MP, Mesotten D, Hermans G, et al. Early versus late parenteral nutrition in critically ill adults. N Engl J Med 2011;365(6):506–17.
24. McCowen KC, Friel C, Sternberg J, et al. Hypocaloric total parenteral nutrition: effectiveness in prevention of hyperglycemia and infectious complications–a randomized clinical trial. Crit Care Med 2000;28(11):3606–11.
25. Briet F, Jeejeebhoy KN. Effect of hypoenergetic feeding and refeeding on muscle and mononuclear cell activities of mitochondrial complexes I–IV in enterally fed rats. Am J Clin Nutr 2001;73(5):975–83.
26. Weijs P, Cynober L, DeLegge M, et al. Proteins and amino acids are fundamental to optimal nutrition support in critically ill patients. Crit Care 2014;18(6):591.
27. Arabi YM, Haddad SH, Tamim HM, et al. Near-target caloric intake in critically ill medical-surgical patients is associated with adverse outcomes. JPEN J Parenter Enteral Nutr 2010;34(3):280–8.
28. Rubinson L, Diette GB, Song X, et al. Low caloric intake is associated with nosocomial bloodstream infections in patients in the medical intensive care unit. Crit Care Med 2004;32(2):350–7.
29. Krishnan JA, Parce PB, Martinez A, et al. Caloric intake in medical ICU patients: consistency of care with guidelines and relationship to clinical outcomes. Chest 2003;124(1):297–305.
30. Dickerson RN, Boschert KJ, Kudsk KA, et al. Hypocaloric enteral tube feeding in critically ill obese patients. Nutrition 2002;18(3):241–6.
31. Heyland DK, Cahill N, Day AG. Optimal amount of calories for critically ill patients: depends on how you slice the cake! Crit Care Med 2011;39(12):2619–26.
32. Arabi YM, Tamim HM, Dhar GS, et al. Permissive underfeeding and intensive insulin therapy in critically ill patients: a randomized controlled trial. Am J Clin Nutr 2011;93(3):569–77.

33. Arabi YM, Aldawood AS, Haddad SH, et al. Permissive underfeeding or standard enteral feeding in critically ill adults. N Engl J Med 2015;372(25):2398–408.
34. Rice TW, Mogan S, Hays MA, et al. Randomized trial of initial trophic versus full-energy enteral nutrition in mechanically ventilated patients with acute respiratory failure. Crit Care Med 2011;39(5):967–74.
35. National Heart, Lung, and Blood Institute Acute Respiratory Distress Syndrome (ARDS) Clinical Trials Network, Rice TW, Wheeler AP, et al. Initial trophic vs full enteral feeding in patients with acute lung injury: the EDEN randomized trial. JAMA 2012;307(8):795–803.
36. Kudsk KA, Croce MA, Fabian TC, et al. Enteral versus parenteral feeding. Effects on septic morbidity after blunt and penetrating abdominal trauma. Ann Surg 1992;215(5):503–11 [discussion: 511–3].
37. Simpson F, Doig GS. Parenteral vs. enteral nutrition in the critically ill patient: a meta-analysis of trials using the intention to treat principle. Intensive Care Med 2005;31(1):12–23.
38. Harvey SE, Segaran E, Leonard R. Trial of the route of early nutritional support in critically ill adults. N Engl J Med 2015;372(5):488–9.
39. Kreymann KG, Berger MM, Deutz NE, et al. ESPEN guidelines on enteral nutrition: intensive care. Clin Nutr 2006;25(2):210–23.
40. Bauer P, Charpentier C, Bouchet C, et al. Parenteral with enteral nutrition in the critically ill. Intensive Care Med 2000;26(7):893–900.
41. Herndon DN, Barrow RE, Stein M, et al. Increased mortality with intravenous supplemental feeding in severely burned patients. J Burn Care Rehabil 1989;10(4):309–13.
42. Casaer MP, Wilmer A, Van den Berghe G. Supplemental parenteral nutrition in critically ill patients. Lancet 2013;381(9879):1715.
43. Doig GS, Simpson F, Sweetman EA, et al. Early parenteral nutrition in critically ill patients with short-term relative contraindications to early enteral nutrition: a randomized controlled trial. JAMA 2013;309(20):2130–8.
44. Heidegger CP, Berger MM, Graf S, et al. Optimisation of energy provision with supplemental parenteral nutrition in critically ill patients: a randomised controlled clinical trial. Lancet 2013;381(9864):385–93.
45. Sax HC, Illig KA, Ryan CK, et al. Low-dose enteral feeding is beneficial during total parenteral nutrition. Am J Surg 1996;171(6):587–90.
46. Yang S, Wu X, Yu W, et al. Early enteral nutrition in critically ill patients with hemodynamic instability: an evidence-based review and practical advice. Nutr Clin Pract 2014;29(1):90–6.
47. Cresci G, Cue J. The patient with circulatory shock: to feed or not to feed? Nutr Clin Pract 2008;23(5):501–9.
48. McClave SA, Chang WK. Feeding the hypotensive patient: does enteral feeding precipitate or protect against ischemic bowel? Nutr Clin Pract 2003;18(4):279–84.
49. Deitch EA. Bacterial translocation of the gut flora. J Trauma 1990;30(12 Suppl):S184–9.
50. Kles KA, Wallig MA, Tappenden KA. Luminal nutrients exacerbate intestinal hypoxia in the hypoperfused jejunum. JPEN J Parenter Enteral Nutr 2001;25(5):246–53.
51. Kazamias P, Kotzampassi K, Koufogiannis D, et al. Influence of enteral nutrition-induced splanchnic hyperemia on the septic origin of splanchnic ischemia. World J Surg 1998;22(1):6–11.
52. Bounous G, Sutherland NG, McArdle AH, et al. The prophylactic use of an "elemental" diet in experimental hemorrhagic shock and intestinal ischemia. Ann Surg 1967;166(3):312–43.

53. Revelly JP, Tappy L, Berger MM, et al. Early metabolic and splanchnic responses to enteral nutrition in postoperative cardiac surgery patients with circulatory compromise. Intensive Care Med 2001;27(3):540–7.
54. Berger MM, Chiolero RL. Enteral nutrition and cardiovascular failure: from myths to clinical practice. JPEN J Parenter Enteral Nutr 2009;33(6):702–9.
55. Funk DJ, Jacobsohn E, Kumar A. The role of venous return in critical illness and shock-part I: physiology. Crit Care Med 2013;41(1):255–62.
56. Rai SS, O'Connor SN, Lange K, et al. Enteral nutrition for patients in septic shock: a retrospective cohort study. Crit Care Resusc 2010;12(3):177–81.
57. Khalid I, Doshi P, DiGiovine B. Early enteral nutrition and outcomes of critically ill patients treated with vasopressors and mechanical ventilation. Am J Crit Care 2010;19(3):261–8.
58. Elke G, Kuhnt E, Ragaller M, et al. Enteral nutrition is associated with improved outcome in patients with severe sepsis. A secondary analysis of the VISEP trial. Med Klin Intensivmed Notfmed 2013;108(3):223–33.
59. Rokyta R Jr, Matejovic M, Krouzecky A, et al. Post-pyloric enteral nutrition in septic patients: effects on hepato-splanchnic hemodynamics and energy status. Intensive Care Med 2004;30(4):714–7.
60. Patel JJ, Kozeniecki M, Biesboer A, et al. Early trophic enteral nutrition is associated with improved outcomes in mechanically ventilated patients with septic shock: a retrospective review. J Intensive Care Med 2014. [Epub ahead of print].

# Gut Motility Issues in Critical Illness

Robert W. Taylor, MD, MCCM*

**KEYWORDS**

- Acute gastrointestinal injury • Gastrointestinal symptoms
- Prevalence of acute gastrointestinal injury • Ileus • Gastrointestinal dysmotility
- Intra-abdominal hypertension

**KEY POINTS**

- Acute gastrointestinal injury (AGI), including delayed gastric emptying, abnormal intestinal motility patterns, and impaired intestinal barrier integrity, is common in critically ill patients.
- Acute AGI may lead to increased morbidity and mortality in critically ill patients.
- This disorder is associated with a wide variety of signs and symptoms and may be difficult to detect, therefore a high index of suspicion is warranted.
- Defects in gastrointestinal motor function, gastrointestinal barrier function, neuroendocrine function, and immune function occur.
- AGI secondary to critical illness may impair the patient's ability to absorb needed nutrients and lead to malnutrition and decreased immune competence.

## INTRODUCTION

Acute gastrointestinal injury (AGI) is both common and potentially deadly.[1–3] The presence of AGI may be occult and its severity may not be immediately apparent to the clinician.

AGI is often manifest by impaired:

- Gastric emptying
- Intestinal motility
- Absorption of fluids, electrolytes, and nutrients
- Mucosal barrier integrity
- Endocrine function
- Immunologic function
- Gut regulatory function

Disclosures: None.

Department of Critical Care Medicine, Mercy Hospital St. Louis, Suite 4006B, St Louis, MO 63141, USA
* Corresponding author.
*E-mail address:* Taylrw@mercy.net

Crit Care Clin 32 (2016) 191–201
http://dx.doi.org/10.1016/j.ccc.2015.11.003 criticalcare.theclinics.com
0749-0704/16/$ – see front matter 

A variety of definitions have been used to describe AGI. This variety has led to clinical confusion and hampered comparison of research across institutions. An international working group of the European Society of Intensive Care Medicine (ESICM) was convened to standardize definitions for AGI and provide current evidence-based understanding of the pathophysiology and management. The results of this working group were published in 2012 and are addressed later.[1]

## GUT COMPONENTS

Gut components include:

- Intestinal epithelium
- Mucosal immune system
- Enteric nervous system
- Gut microflora

Dysfunction or failure of any of these components leads to AGI. The dysfunction may be isolated to 1 area of the gastrointestinal (GI) tract or it may be generalized.

## SIGNS AND SYMPTOMS OF ACUTE GASTROINTESTINAL INJURY

Signs and symptoms associated with AGI are common[3–5] and include:

- Nausea and vomiting
- Absent or abnormal bowel sounds
- Abdominal distention
- Diarrhea
- Constipation
- Inability to enterally feed patients
- GI hemorrhage

## GASTROINTESTINAL BLEEDING

GI bleeding to at least some extent is commonly seen in critically ill patients, with most showing endoscopic evidence of mucosal erosion secondary to mucosal stress.[6] This condition most commonly presents as:

- Hematemesis
- Coffee ground emesis
- Blood in nasogastric tube
- Melena

Although less common, hemodynamically significant GI hemorrhage presenting as bright red blood from the upper or lower GI tract has potentially lethal consequences and occurs often enough in critically ill patients to warrant careful attention.

## ISCHEMIA-REPERFUSION INJURY

Resuscitation of circulatory shock may lead to an enterocyte villous ischemia-reperfusion injury characterized by[7,8]:

- Epithelial cell disruption
- Diminished villous height
- Mucosal cell necrosis
- Accelerated apoptosis
- Increased enterocyte shedding

- Compromise of gut barrier function
- Water, electrolyte, and nutrient malabsorption
- Feeding intolerance
- Alternated secretion of:
  - Ions
  - Regulatory molecules
  - Amino acids
  - Protective mucus
- Derangement of GI immunologic function
- Abnormal interaction of GI microflora with gut mucosa

## GASTROINTESTINAL DYSMOTILITY

Most critical illnesses cause significant GI dysmotility and many of the signs and symptoms of AGI are directly linked to abnormal motility.

Upper GI motility disorders commonly include[9,10]:

- Decreased gastroesophageal sphincter tone
- Increased gastroesophageal reflux
- Delayed gastric emptying with high residual volumes
- Abnormal pyloric sphincter tone
- Abnormal (retrograde) duodenal contraction waves

Beyond the duodenum the small bowel does not seem to be involved to the same extent as the upper GI tract. Small bowel transit time seems to be largely unaffected by critical illness.[11] Colonic motility disorders are common and lead to both diarrhea and constipation. Increased colonic transit time is commonly seen in postoperative patients (intra-abdominal procedures, narcotics). Alternatively, reduced colonic transit time leading to diarrhea is seen in more than 50% of intensive care unit (ICU) patients.[12–14]

Numerous neuroendocrine and immune pathways, molecules, and mediators are involved in normal gastrointestinal physiology. Although precise pathophysiologic mechanisms are still under investigation it is clear that disruption of these pathways commonly leads to GI dysmotility.

Motor function in the upper GI tract is influenced by central and local GI neuroendocrine mechanisms that provide rhythmic and coordinated GI smooth muscle peristalsis. When sympathetic and parasympathetic nervous activity is disrupted dysmotility is often a consequence.[15] Sympathetic blockade is associated with abnormally increased GI motility, whereas parasympathetic blockade (vagus) is associated with delayed gastric emptying.[16]

Poor gut contractility and slow intestinal transit times in critically patients are common and involve overproduction and secretion of inhibitory neurotransmitters, including[17]:

- Nitric oxide
- Vasoactive intestinal peptide
- Tachykinins
- Neurokinins

Common ICU disorders and treatments that lead to dysmotility include[16,18,19]:

- Hyperglycemia or hypoglycemia
- Hypokalemia
- Hypophosphatemia

- Intra-abdominal hypertension
- Intracranial hypertension
- Positive pressure mechanical ventilation
- Opioid use
- Use of nonopioid sedatives
- Intravenous catecholamines
- Intra-abdominal hypertension
- Intraoperative intestinal manipulation
- Hemorrhage

Diarrhea in the critically ill is common, but is probably not often directly related to reduced intestinal transit times; it is more closely associated with antibiotic use, osmolar effect of tube feeding, and/or hypoalbuminemia.

Overgrowth of pathogenic bacteria occurs commonly in critically ill patients and, in turn, may lead to a vicious cycle with[20,21]:

- Further altered mucosal barrier integrity
- Altered gut motility
- Water, electrolyte, and nutrient malabsorption
- Diarrhea

## MOTOR FUNCTION OF THE PROXIMAL GASTROINTESTINAL TRACT

Peristalsis in the upper GI tract is under both central and enteric neuroendocrine control. Heightened sympathetic nervous system activity and/or catecholamine administration may impede gastric emptying and slow peristalsis.[15] In contrast, the sympathetic blockade seen with epidural anesthesia is associated with an increase in GI motility.[18]

Normal parasympathetic (vagal) activity is critical for normal GI tract motility. Vagal inhibition impedes gastric emptying.[9] Slowed intestinal transit times associated with impaired peristalsis is common in the critically ill and involves secretion of inhibitory neurotransmitters such as nitric oxide, vasoactive intestinal peptide, substance P, and neurokinins.[17] Accelerated peristalsis is therefore not a common cause of diarrhea, but a variety of clinical factors may lead to diarrhea, including hypoalbuminemia and use of antibiotics that alter normal gut flora and disturb normal peristalsis.[21]

Abnormalities in secretion of gastrointestinal hormones are also common in critical illness. Increased secretion of cholecystokinin and peptide YY is common in critical illness and is associated with delayed gastric emptying.[22] Similarly, high plasma motilin levels are seen in critically ill patients in response to feeding, which, in turn, is associated with delayed gastric emptying.[23]

Proinflammatory cytokine levels are commonly increased in the critically ill. This increase often leads to abnormal GI tract barrier function. Experimental models suggest that increased secretion of proinflammatory cytokines also plays an important role in modulating GI tract neuromuscular function. The muscularis layer of the intestinal wall is adversely affected by proinflammatory cytokines, leading to alteration in smooth muscle ion channels[24] and impaired contractility. Disordered peristalsis may also be modulated by cytokine-induced alteration in spinal afferent neurons.

## GASTROINTESTINAL TRACT BARRIER DYSFUNCTION

Interleukin-6 and tumor necrosis factor-alpha, are central figures in maintenance of GI tract barrier integrity.[25] Occludin and zona occludens protein-1 are membrane-associated proteins and regulate GI tract cellular tight junctions.[26] As proinflammatory cytokines, interleukin-6 and tumor necrosis factor-alpha induce a marked reduction in intestinal levels of occludin and zona occludens protein-1, leading to loss of tight junctions and GI tract barrier dysfunction.

Circulatory shock and resuscitation leads to GI tract ischemia-reperfusion injury. Loss of small bowel barrier function is common. Pathologic changes are seen, such as epithelial cell necrosis and apoptosis and relaxation of GI tract epithelial tight junctions.[26] Crystalloid resuscitation is associated with more pronounced GI tract barrier dysfunction than colloid resuscitation, although a difference in clinical outcome has not been established.[27,28]

GI tract mucus is an important vehicle for mucin-associated regeneration and repair, which is necessary for maintenance of GI tract barrier integrity.[29] Ischemia-reperfusion injury is associated with a change in GI mucus quality leading to increased GI tract barrier permeability.[13]

Pathologic GI tract flora adversely interacts with GI tract epithelium causing[20,30]:

- Enhanced inflammatory processes
- Disruption of tight junctions
- GI epithelial cell loss
- Reduction in stool content of organic acids that act as fuel for regeneration of mucosal cells and stimulate mucin production

Enteral supplementation of critically ill patients with probiotic bacteria is attractive from a theoretic perspective and is under investigation. In a murine model of colitis, patients treated with probiotics showed reduced GI tract mucosal inflammation and improved barrier function.[31–33] Patients with trauma given enteral probiotics have shown a reduction in inflammatory cytokine secretion with improvement in intestinal barrier function.[32] Besselink and colleagues[34] raised a note of caution when they reported an increase in mortality in patients with severe acute pancreatitis treated with probiotics.

Other clinical conditions have been reported to worsen GI tract barrier leak, including[35]:

- Sepsis, severe sepsis, and septic shock
- Severe acute pancreatitis
- Jaundice
- Inflammatory bowel disease
- Intraoperative manipulation of bowel

Many of the mechanisms listed earlier work in concert to cause GI tract barrier dysfunction.

## INCREASED MORBIDITY AND MORTALITY WITH ACUTE GASTROINTESTINAL INJURY

The increased morbidity and mortality associated with AGI are most likely caused by decreased nutrient absorption and increased risk of infection.

### *Nutritional Deficits*

Gastric stasis is likely the most common cause of enteral feeding intolerance and has been reported to occur in as many as 35% of enterally fed patients in the ICU.[7,8] Although the precise definition of feeding intolerance is under debate, it is clear that critically ill patients often receive only a portion (40%–60%) of nutritional requirements while receiving tube feedings.[36,37] Early initiation of enteral feeding may help.

Rodriguez and colleagues[38] reported improvement in gastric emptying if enteral feedings were started within 6 hours of the time of burn injury.

Small bowel dysfunction also plays a role in malabsorption of nutrients. Normal small bowel peristalsis is important for nutrient absorption. When feeding is delayed, fasting state motility patterns may lead to unabsorbed nutrients being dumped into the large intestine with resultant diarrhea.[39] Small bowel bacterial overgrowth also leads to diarrhea. Malnutrition in the critically ill is associated with increased morbidity and mortality, including increased risk of GI tract–associated infection.

### *Gastrointestinal Tract–associated Infection*

Malnutrition in the critically ill is associated with increased morbidity and mortality, including an increased risk of GI tract–associated infection.[40,41] The most common GI tract–associated infections are aspiration with ventilator-associated pneumonia and GI tract–associated sepsis.

### *Aspiration of Enteral Feeding*

A concern over the possibility of aspiration of enteral feedings is central in many ICUs. Limiting enteral feeding to reduce the risk of aspiration can lead to malnutrition and increase the risk of infection. In contrast, feeding beyond the limit of the stomach and upper small bowel capability can lead to regurgitation and aspiration of stomach and small bowel contents, with attendant worsening of pulmonary function and risk of pulmonary infection.

Many ICUs monitor gastric residual volume as an indicator of impending aspiration. Controversy exists as to what volume of residual gastric contents should be considered dangerous. From 200 to 500 mL is a commonly quoted range but there is a distinct absence of evidence to support this contention. When high residual volume alone is used to halt or terminate enteral feeding significant underfeeding may occur. This underfeeding in turn is associated with an increased risk of nosocomial infection, including pneumonia. High residual volumes alone have never been shown to predict aspiration pneumonia. However, high gastric residual volumes in the setting of vomiting have been associated with nosocomial pneumonia, prolonged ICU stays, and increased mortality.[40]

### *The Gut Hypothesis of Sepsis*

Dysfunctional GI tract motor activity in the critically ill may impair elimination of intestinal contents with attendant prolonged exposure to both pathologic microorganisms and their antigenic products.[41] Prolonged contact of these pathogens in the setting of impaired GI tract barrier function has been described as the "motor of critical illness."[42] Recent evidence indicates that infectious complications and mortality are significantly increased in patients with the systemic inflammatory response syndrome, who have reduced normal flora within the GI tract.[41] Preliminary studies support a reduction in infectious complications and a reduction in ventilator-associated pneumonia when probiotics were used.[43]

## STANDARDIZING DEFINITIONS/TREATMENT RECOMMENDATIONS

As mentioned earlier, a variety of definitions have been used to describe AGI, which has led to clinical confusion and hampered comparison of research across institutions. An international working group of the ESICM suggested standardized definitions for AGI in hopes of improving communication and to provide current evidence-based

**Table 1**
**AGI grade, examples, and treatment recommendations**

| AGI Grade | Example | Treatment Considerations |
|---|---|---|
| I | Postoperative nausea and/or vomiting during the first days after abdominal surgery, postoperative absence of bowel sounds, diminished bowel motility in the early phase of shock | The general condition is usually improving and specific interventions for GI symptoms are not needed, except the replacement of fluid requirements by intravenous infusions. Early enteral feeding, started within 24–48 h after the injury, is recommended. The use of drugs impairing GI motility (eg, catecholamines, opioids) has to be limited whenever possible |
| II | Gastroparesis with high gastric residuals or reflux, paralysis of the lower GI tract, diarrhea, IAH grade I (IAP 12–15 mm Hg), visible blood in gastric content or stool. Feeding intolerance is present if at least 20 kcal/kg/d via enteral route cannot be reached within 72 h of feeding attempt | Measures to treat the condition and to prevent the progression to GI failure need to be undertaken (eg, treatment of intra-abdominal hypertension); or measures to restore the motility function of the GI tract, such as prokinetic therapy. Enteral feeding should be started or continued; in cases of high gastric residuals/reflux or feeding intolerance, regular challenges with small amounts of EN should be regularly considered. In patients with gastroparesis, initiation of postpyloric feeding should be considered in this state, when prokinetic therapy is not effective |
| III | Despite treatment, feeding intolerance persists: high gastric residuals, persisting GI paralysis, occurrence or worsening of bowel dilatation, progression of IAH to grade II (IAP 15–20 mm Hg), low APP (<60 mm Hg). Feeding intolerance is present and possibly associated with persistence or worsening of MODS | Measures to prevent worsening of GI failure are warranted (eg, monitoring and targeted treatment of IAH). Presence of undiagnosed abdominal problem (cholecystitis, peritonitis, bowel ischemia) should be excluded. The medications promoting GI paralysis should be discontinued as far as possible. Early parenteral feeding (within the first 7 d of ICU stay) supplementary to insufficient enteral nutrition is associated with higher incidence of hospital infections and should be avoided. Challenges with small amounts of EN should be regularly considered |
| IV | Bowel ischemia with necrosis, GI bleeding leading to hemorrhagic shock, Ogilvie syndrome, ACS requiring decompression | Condition requires laparotomy or other emergency interventions (eg, colonoscopy for colonic decompression) for lifesaving indications |

*Abbreviations:* ACS, abdominal compartment syndrome; APP, abdominal perfusion pressure; EN, enteral nutrition; IAH, intra-abdominal hypertension; IAP, intra-abdominal pressure.

*Data from* Refs.[1,43–58]

understanding of the pathophysiology and management. The results of this working group were published in 2012.[1] The report focuses on 4 grades of AGI:

- AGI grade I (risk of developing GI dysfunction or failure): the function of the GI tract is partially impaired, expressed as GI symptoms related to a known cause and perceived as transient.
- AGI grade II (gastrointestinal dysfunction): the GI tract is not able to perform digestion and absorption adequately to satisfy the nutrient and fluid requirements of the body. There are no changes in general condition of the patient related to GI problems.
- AGI grade III (gastrointestinal failure): loss of GI function, in which restoration of GI function is not achieved despite interventions, and the general condition is not improving.
- AGI grade IV (gastrointestinal failure with severe impact on distant organ function): AGI has progressed to become directly and immediately life threatening, with worsening of Multiple organ dysfunction syndrome (MODS) and shock. Rationale Situation when AGI has led to an acute critical deterioration of the general condition of the patient with distant organ dysfunction.

Clinical examples for AGI grade and treatment recommendations are shown in **Table 1**.

## SUMMARY

AGI is both common and potentially deadly. The signs and symptoms are varied and may include nausea, vomiting, abnormal bowel sounds, abdominal distention and pain, diarrhea, constipation, inability to tolerate enteral feeding, and GI hemorrhage. The presence of AGI may be occult and its severity initially difficult to determine. Resuscitation from circulatory shock may be associated with morphologic changes in GI epithelium that lead to multiple forms of GI disorder. GI motor dysfunction, GI barrier dysfunction, neuroendocrine dysfunction, and immune dysfunction occur. Absorption of nutrients is often impaired. Aspiration pneumonia and propagation of critical illness, including systemic inflammatory response syndrome, severe sepsis, and septic shock, are potential concerns with AGI. Treatment depends on the severity of AGI and the specific pathophysiologic defect (see **Table 1**).

## REFERENCES


1. Blaser AR, Malbrain MLNG, Fruhwald S, et al. Gastrointestinal function in intensive care patients: terminology, definitions and management. Recommendations of the ESICM working group on abdominal problems. Intensive Care Med 2012; 38:384–94.
2. Rombeau JL, Takala J. Summary of round table conference: gut dysfunction in critical illness. Intensive Care Med 1997;23:476–9.
3. Hill LT. Gut dysfunction in the critically ill – mechanisms and clinical implications. S Afr J Crit Care 2013;29:11–5.
4. Reintam A, Parm P, Kitus R, et al. Gastrointestinal symptoms in intensive care patients. Acta Anaesthesiol Scand 2009;53:318–24.
5. Hill LT, Hill B, Miller M, et al. The effect of intra-abdominal hypertension on gastrointestinal function. South African Journal of Critical Care 2011;27:12–9.
6. Duerkson DR. Stress-related mucosal disease in critically ill patients. Best Pract Res Clin Gastroenterol 2003;17:327–44.

7. Rupani B, Caputo FJ, Watkins AC, et al. Relationship between disruption of the unstirred mucus layer and intestinal restitution in loss of gut barrier function after trauma hemorrhagic shock. Surgery 2007;141:481–9.
8. Derikx JP, Matthijsen RA, de Bruine AP, et al. A new model to study intestinal ischemia reperfusion damage in man. J Surg Res 2011;166:222–6.
9. Nguyen NQ, Ng MP, Chapman M, et al. The impact of admission diagnosis on gastric emptying in critically ill patients. Crit Care 2007;11:R16.
10. Montejo JC. Enteral nutrition-related gastrointestinal complications in critically ill patients: a multicenter study: the Nutritional and Metabolic Working Group of the Spanish Society of Intensive Care Medicine and Coronary Units. Crit Care Med 1999;27:1447–53.
11. Montejo JC, Grau T, Acosta J, et al, For the Nutritional and Metabolic Working Group of the Spanish Society of Intensive Care Medicine and Coronary Units. Multicenter, prospective, randomized, single-blind study comparing the efficacy and gastrointestinal complications of early jejunal feeding with early gastric feeding in critically ill patients. Crit Care Med 2002;30:796–800.
12. Rauch S, Krueger K, Turan A, et al. Determining small intestinal transit time and pathomorphology in critically ill patients using video capsule technology. Intensive Care Med 2009;35:1054–9.
13. Nguyen NQ, Fraser RJ, Bryant LK, et al. Diminished functional association between proximal and distal gastric motility in critically ill patients. Intensive Care Med 2008;34:1246–55.
14. Tournadre JP, Barclay M, Fraser R, et al. Small intestinal motor patterns in critically ill patients after major abdominal surgery. Am J Gastroenterol 2001;96: 2418–26.
15. Fukudo H, Tsuchida D, Koda K, et al. Inhibition of sympathetic pathways restores postoperative ileus in the upper and lower gastrointestinal tract. J Gastroenterol Hepatol 2007;2:1293–9.
16. Kariv Y, Wang W, Senagore AJ, et al. Multivariate analysis of factors associated with hospital readmission after intestinal surgery. Am J Surg 2006;191:364–71.
17. Holzer P, Holzer-Petsche U. Tachykinins in the gut. Part 1. Expression, release and motor function. Pharmacol Ther 1997;73:173–217.
18. Liu SS, Wong CL. Effect of postoperative analgesia on major postoperative complications: a systematic update of the evidence. Anesth Analg 2007;104(3): 689–702.
19. Mutlu GM, Mutlu EA, Factor P. Prevention and treatment of gastrointestinal complications in patients on mechanical ventilation. Am J Respir Med 2003;2: 395–411.
20. Shimizu K, Ogura H, Goto M, et al. Altered gut flora and environment in patients with severe SIRS. J Trauma 2006;60:126–33.
21. Husebye E, Hellstrom PM, Midtvedt T. Intestinal microflora stimulates myoelectric activity of rat small intestine by promoting cyclic initiation and aboral propagation of migrating myoelectric complex. Dig Dis Sci 1994;39:946–56.
22. Nguyen N, Chapman M, Fraser R, et al. Feed intolerance in critical illness is associated with increased basal and nutrient-stimulated plasma cholecystokinin concentrations. Crit Care Med 2007;35:82–8.
23. Nguyen NF, Bryant R, Burgstad L, et al. Abnormalities in plasma motilin response to small intestinal nutrient stimulation in critically ill patients. Gastroenterology 2010;138 [abstract: S405].
24. Akbarli H, Hawkins EG, Ross GR, et al. Ion channel remodeling in gastrointestinal inflammation. Neurogastroenterol Motil 2010;22:1045–55.

25. Spindler-Vesel A, Wraber B, Vovk I, et al. Intestinal permeability and cytokine inflammatory response in multiply injured patients. J Interferon Cytokine Res 2006;26:771–6.
26. Han X, Fink MP, Delude RL. Proinflammatory cytokines cause NO-dependent and independent changes in expression and localization of tight junction proteins in intestinal epithelial cells. Shock 2002;19:229–37.
27. Vega D, Badami CD, Caputo FJ, et al. The influence of the type of resuscitation fluid on gut injury and distant organ injury in a rat model of trauma/hemorrhagic shock. J Trauma 2008;65:409–14.
28. Finfer S, Bellomo N, Boyce N, et al. A comparison of albumin and saline for fluid resuscitation in the intensive care unit. N Engl J Med 2004;350:2247–56.
29. Higuchi A, Wu R, Zhou M, et al. Gut hyper permeability after ischemia and reperfusion: attenuation with adrenomedullin and its binding protein treatment. Int J Clin Exp Pathol 2008;1:409–18.
30. Cario E, Gerken G, Podolsky DK. Toll-like receptor 2 controls mucosal inflammation by regulating epithelial barrier function. Gastroenterology 2007;132:1359–74.
31. Mennigen R, Nolte K, Rijcken E, et al. Probiotic mixture VSL#3 protects the epithelial barrier by maintaining tight junction protein expression and preventing apoptosis in a murine model of colitis. Am J Physiol Gastrointest Liver Physiol 2009;296:1140–9.
32. Giamarellos-Bourboulis EJ, Bengmark S, Kanellakopoulou K, et al. Pro- and synbiotics to control inflammation and infection in patients with multiple injuries. J Trauma 2009;67:815–21.
33. Peng LY, Li Z, Green RS, et al. Butyrate enhances the intestinal barrier by facilitating tight junction assembly via activation of AMP activated protein kinase in Caco-2 cell monolayers. J Nutr 2009;139:1619–25.
34. Besselink MG, van Santvoort HC, Buskens E, et al. Probiotic prophylaxis in patients with predicted severe acute pancreatitis: a randomised, double-blind, placebo-controlled trial. Ned Tijdschr Geneeskd 2008;152:685–96.
35. Matejovic M, Krouzecky A, Rohyta R, et al. Effects of intestinal surgery on pulmonary, glomerular, and intestinal permeability, and its relation to the hemodynamics and oxidative stress. Surg Today 2004;34:24–31.
36. Poulard F, Dimet J, Martin-Lefevre L, et al. Impact of not measuring residual gastric volume in mechanically ventilated patients receiving early enteral feeding: a prospective before-after study. JPEN J Parenter Enteral Nutr 2010;34:125–30.
37. Heyland DK, Cahill NE, Dhaliwal R, et al. Impact of enteral feeding protocols on enteral nutrition delivery: results of a multicenter observational study. JPEN J Parenter Enteral Nutr 2010;34:675–84.
38. Rodriguez NA, Jeschke MG, Williams FN, et al. Nutrition in burns: Galveston contributions. JPEN J Parenter Enteral Nutr 2011;36:704.
39. Deane AM, Summers MJ, Zaknic AV, et al. Glucose absorption and small intestinal transit in critical illness. Crit Care Med 2011;39:1282–8.
40. Metheny NA, Schallom L, Oliver DA, et al. Gastric residual volume and aspiration in critically ill patients receiving gastric feedings. Am J Crit Care 2008;17:512–9.
41. Shimizu K, Ogura H, Hamasaki T, et al. Altered gut flora are associated with septic complications and death in critically ill patients with systemic inflammatory response syndrome. Dig Dis Sci 2011;56:1171–7.
42. Clark JA, Coopersmith CM. Intestinal crosstalk – a new paradigm for understanding the gut as the "motor" of critical illness. Shock 2007;28:384–93.
43. Morrow LE, Kollef MH, Casale TB. Probiotic prophylaxis of ventilator-associated pneumonia: a blinded, randomized, controlled trial. Am J Respir Crit Care Med 2010;182:1058–64.

44. Alverdy JC, Change EB. The re-emerging role of intestinal microflora in critical illness and inflammation: why the gut hypothesis of sepsis syndrome will not go away. J Leukoc Biol 2008;83:461–6.
45. Piton G, Manzon C, Cypriant B, et al. Acute intestinal failure in critically ill patients: is plasma citrulline the right marker? Intensive Care Med 2011;37:911–7.
46. Doig GS, Heighes PT, Simpson F, et al. Early enteral nutrition, provided within 24 h of injury or intensive care unit admission, significantly reduces mortality in critically ill patients: a meta-analysis of randomized controlled trials. Intensive Care Med 2007;35:2018–27.
47. Antonelli M, Azoulay E, Bonten M, et al. Year in review in intensive care medicine 2009: I. Pneumonia and infections, sepsis, outcome, acute renal failure and acid base, nutrition and glycemic control. Intensive Care Med 2009;36:196–209.
48. Fruhwald S, Scheidl S, Toller W, et al. Low potential of dobutamine and dopexamine to block intestinal peristalsis as compared with other catecholamines. Crit Care Med 2000;28:2893–7.
49. Nguyen NQ, Chapman MJ, Fraser RJ, et al. The effects of sedation on gastric emptying and intra-gastric meal distribution in critical illness. Intensive Care Med 2007;34:454–60.
50. Fruhwald S, Herk E, Petnehazy T, et al. Sufentanil potentiates the inhibitory effect of epinephrine on intestinal motility. Intensive Care Med 2002;28:74–80.
51. McArthur CJ, Gin T, McLaren IM, et al. Gastric emptying following brain injury: effects of choice of sedation and intracranial pressure. Intensive Care Med 1995; 21:573–6.
52. Cheatham ML, Malbrain ML, Kirkpatrick A, et al. Results from the international conference of experts on intra-abdominal hypertension and abdominal compartment syndrome. II. Recommendations. Intensive Care Med 2007;33:951–62.
53. Fruhwald S, Holzer P, Metzler H. Gastrointestinal motility in acute illness. Wien Klin Wochenschr 2008;120:6–17.
54. Herbert MK, Holzer P. Standardized concept for the treatment of gastrointestinal dysmotility in critically ill patients—current status and future concepts. Clin Nutr 2008;27:25–41.
55. Nguyen NQ, Chapman M, Fraser RJ, et al. Prokinetic therapy for feed intolerance in critical illness: 1 drug or two? Crit Care Med 2007;35:2561–7.
56. Casaer MP, Mesotten D, Hermans G, et al. Early versus late parenteral nutrition in critically ill adults. N Engl J Med 2011;365:506–17.
57. Saunders MD, Kimmey MB. Systematic review: acute colonic pseudo-obstruction. Aliment Pharmacol Ther 2005;22:917–25.
58. De Giorgio R, Barbara G, Stanghellini V, et al. Review article: the pharmacological treatment of acute colonic pseudo-obstruction. Aliment Pharmacol Ther 2001;15: 1717–27.

# The Gut as the Motor of Multiple Organ Dysfunction in Critical Illness

Nathan J. Klingensmith, MD, Craig M. Coopersmith, MD*

**KEYWORDS**

• Sepsis • MODS • Gut • Intestine • Critical illness

**KEY POINTS**

- The gut is composed of an epithelium, adaptive immune system, and microbiome. Each plays a crucial role in the maintenance of health and the pathophysiology of critical illness.
- Toxic mediators travel through mesenteric lymphatics, causing remote inflammatory injury. Preclinical trials have demonstrated that ligation of the lymph duct can prevent lung injury caused by gut-derived factors.
- Gut integrity is compromised in critical illness with increases in apoptosis and permeability. Multiple preclinical studies have demonstrated that targeting gut epithelial integrity results in improved survival in critical illness.
- The microbiome can alter its behavior based on environmental cues. Preventing bacteria from becoming virulent or reprogramming them to a nonvirulent phenotype may revolutionize the treatment of gut-derived sepsis.
- Outside of enteral nutrition, no treatment targeting the gut is currently widely used in the intensive care unit. Multiple techniques for modulating the microbiome are of potential interest as therapeutics.

## OVERVIEW

The gut has been hypothesized to be the motor of multiple organ dysfunction syndrome (MODS) for the past quarter century.[1–3] Whereas initial theories of gut and critical illness suggested that hyperpermeability resulted in bacterial translocation into the systemic circulation, the reality is significantly more complex than was hypothesized originally. All elements of the gut—the epithelium, the immune system, and the microbiome—are impacted by critical illness and can, in turn, propagate a pathologic host

---

This work was supported by funding from the National Institutes of Health (GM104323, GM095442, GM072808, GM109779 and GM113228).
Department of Surgery, Emory Critical Care Center, Emory University School of Medicine, Atlanta, GA, USA
* Corresponding author. 101 Woodruff Circle, Suite WMB 5105, Atlanta, GA 30322.
*E-mail address:* cmcoop3@emory.edu

Crit Care Clin 32 (2016) 203–212
http://dx.doi.org/10.1016/j.ccc.2015.11.004 criticalcare.theclinics.com
0749-0704/16/$ – see front matter 

response. Further, alterations in the gut can lead to both local and distant insults, via alterations in homeostatic processes and defense mechanisms as well as release of toxic mediators into both the mesenteric lymph and the systemic circulation. Although considerable effort has been put into directly targeting the gut for therapeutic gain in critical illness, the results to date have been modest. This review focuses on the cellular and molecular underpinnings of how the gut functions as the motor of MODS, as well as clinical ways in which the gut can, at least in part, be potentially manipulated for therapeutic gain.

## THE GUT IN HEALTH

### *Epithelium*

The gut contains a single layer epithelium with a myriad of important functions. It provides a large surface area—estimated to be approximately 32 $m^2$ or one-half the size of a badminton court[4]—for use in nutrient absorption and preventing entrance of pathogens from its lumen. Microscopically, the gut is in a state of constant renewal from the multipotent stem cells near the crypt base. These give rise to daughter cells, which then give rise to 4 major intestinal cell types: (a) enterocytes, which absorb nutrients and make up greater than 90% of intestinal epithelial cells, (b) mucus-producing goblet cells, (c) hormone-producing enteroendocrine cells, and (d) defensin-producing Paneth cells that protect intestinal stems cells and play a role in intestine–microbiota interactions.[5] Unlike other cells in the gut that migrate upward along the villus, Paneth cells migrate downward toward the crypt base. The journey from cell birth, differentiation, and migration along the villus to cell loss via either apoptosis or luminal sloughing of intact cells takes only 5 to 7 days in a healthy human.

### *Immune System*

The intestine is the largest lymphoid organ of the body.[6] It contains 4 immune cell compartments: Peyer's patches, the lamina propria, mesenteric lymph nodes, and intraepithelial lymphocytes. Peyer's patches come in contact with luminal antigens and direct antigen-presenting cells to the mesenteric lymph nodes. This sets off the immune differentiation of T and B cells in the draining nodes. The highly complicated gut mucosal immune system plays a myriad of roles in host defense including (but not limited to) antigen recognition, presentation, amplification of antigen-specific response, and production of cytokines and chemokines.[7]

### *Microbiome*

There are 10 times more bacterial cells in a human than host cells—100 trillion bacteria to 10 trillion human cells.[8] Under normal conditions, there is a well-tolerated symbiotic relationship between the human host and its microbiome, which has a robust diversity, with the predominant species being *Bacteroides* and *Firmicutes*. With the recent explosion in our (still nascent) understanding of the microbiome, it has become apparent that the diversity of an individual's microbiota depends on a wide variety of factors starting from the type of birth they underwent (vaginal or Cesarean section) to the diet they eat to their age to even the pets they have.[9]

## PRECLINICAL INSIGHTS INTO THE ROLE OF THE GUT AS THE MOTOR OF MULTIPLE ORGAN DYSFUNCTION SYNDROME

### *The Gut Lymph Hypothesis*

Given the overwhelming number of bacteria that reside in the intestine, the initial hypothesis for why the gut is the motor of MODS was whole bacteria translocation that spread via portal circulation. Although bacterial translocation clearly occurs in some preclinical models of critical illness,[10] human data have generally remained inconclusive or not supportive of this as a common phenomenon seen in critically ill patients, although it likely occurs in select pathophysiologic conditions.[11,12] A search for how intestine-derived mediators caused distant injury led to the gut–lymph hypothesis. This theory postulates that toxic mediators from the gut travel through mesenteric lymphatics toward the lung where they cause remote injury. Several lines of investigation support the importance of the gut-derived lymph as being physiologically important. When the mesenteric lymph duct is ligated in multiple models of critical illness, lung injury and neutrophil activation are abrogated or prevented and, importantly, mortality is diminished or prevented.[13,14] Additionally, when mesenteric lymph from rats undergoing trauma/hemorrhagic shock is injected into nonmanipulated rats, the rats receiving the injection develop lung injury similar to shock rats.[15] Of note, gut-derived lymph typically does not contain intact bacteria, endotoxin, or cytokines but rather contains protein or lipid factors that stimulate Toll-like receptor 4, leading to activation of inflammatory neutrophils in the lung. Although not a part of the gut–lymph hypothesis, it has also been shown that gut-specific deletion of Mttp (a protein required for chylomicron assembly) improves survival in septic mice subjected to *Pseudomonas aeruginosa* pneumonia,[16] although aged animals with the identical genetic knockout have lower survival when subjected to the same insult.[17]

### *Apoptosis*

Cell death via apoptosis is an evolutionarily conserved process that is important for normal development and function. However, gut epithelial apoptosis seems to be detrimental after the onset of sepsis. Both preclinical mouse models of sepsis and autopsy studies of patients who died in the intensive care unit (ICU) demonstrate a marked upregulation in gut epithelial apoptosis compared with those who die without sepsis.[18,19] Gut-specific overexpression of the antiapoptotic protein Bcl-2 has been shown to decrease sepsis-induced intestinal epithelial apoptosis and importantly improve survival in murine models of both cecal ligation and puncture and *P aeruginosa* pneumonia.[20,21] Notably, this beneficial effect of Bcl-2 overexpression is abrogated in septic mice with cancer, suggesting that alterations in the host response caused by comorbidities can impact gut apoptosis.[22]

There is evidence that cross-talk exists between the intestinal epithelium and immune system in sepsis that results in changes in gut epithelial apoptosis. Although the presence or absence of lymphocytes does not impact gut epithelial apoptosis under basal conditions, sepsis-induced gut epithelial apoptosis is significantly higher in $Rag^{-/-}$ mice (which lack lymphocytes) than wild-type mice, suggesting that lymphocytes play an antiapoptotic role in the gut epithelium that is, unmasked in sepsis.[23] Subset analysis demonstrates that $CD4^+$ T cells are responsible for the antiapoptotic effect of the adaptive immune system on the gut epithelium. In addition, when Bcl-2 is overexpressed in myeloid cells, there is a decrease in the amount of gut epithelial apoptosis after sepsis, in addition to improved survival.[24]

### *Hyperpermeability*

The intestinal epithelium consists of only a single layer of cells that is responsible for maintaining a permaselective barrier that, in a simplistic description, is charged with keeping out the bad and letting in the good. It performs these functions via cell–cell intramembrane protein interactions within the tight junction.[25] There are several families of intramembrane proteins (claudins, occludin, tricellulin, junctional adhesion molecule), as well as intracellular connector proteins (zonula occludins, myosin light chain) that link the tight junction to the intracellular cytoskeleton and allow for modulation of the space.[26,27] Alteration of this space can lead to changes in intestinal permeability, and there is significant evidence that intestinal permeability is increased after sepsis and MODS.[28,29]

There is increasing preclinical evidence that targeting tight junctions directly or indirectly might have beneficial effects in critical illness. When myosin light chain kinase is activated, it phosphorylates the myosin light chain causing contraction of the cytoskeleton, increasing the intercellular space and thereby increasing permeability. Inhibiting myosin light chain kinase in mice in the setting of binge alcohol ingestion and burn injury decreases bacterial translocation and intestinal cytokine production to levels seen in sham animals, associated with a prevention in injury-induced alterations in tight junction expression and localization.[30,31] A broader strategy involves targeting global intestinal integrity. Epidermal growth factor is a cytoprotective peptide that exhibits trophic and healing effects on the intestinal mucosa. When mice are given systemic epidermal growth factor after the onset of either cecal ligation and puncture or *P aeruginosa* pneumonia, they have improved or normalized permeability, apoptosis, proliferation, and villus length. Importantly, this is associated with a significant improvement in survival, even if the drug is initiated 24 hours after the onset of sepsis.[32,33] This improvement in survival seems to be mediated through the gut as transgenic mice with enterocyte-specific overexpression of epidermal growth factor have the same improvement in intestinal integrity and survival after sepsis as those that receive systemic epidermal growth factor.[34]

### *Altering the Microbiome*

There is increasing recognition that microbes are not inherently good or bad, but rather alter their behavior based on their environment. Bacteria that are present in someone's healthy microbiome for decades can became virulent if environmental cues suggest an advantage to them. Further, simply the presence of bacteria that can cause fatal disease does not inherently implicate them as being pathologic. For example, *P aeruginosa* injected into the cecum of mice undergoing a sham operation and subsequently removed can be injected into the peritoneum of a control mouse without causing any disease. In contrast, if *P aeruginosa* is injected in the cecum of mice subjected to a nonlethal partial hepatectomy and subsequently removed and injected into a control mouse peritoneum, the resulting mortality is 100%.[35] The ability of bacteria to sense host stress, their own environment, and surrounding bacterial density and alter their virulence in response has profound clinical implications.[36,37] This is because microbial identification without attention to its virulence may not be sufficient for treating critically ill patients while the simple presence of bacteria is not inherently harmful. In addition, virulent bacteria can potentially cause MODS without systemic dissemination. Thus, a potential complementary approach to improving the antibiotic pipeline and preventing antimicrobial resistance is to prevent bacteria from becoming virulent or reprogramming them to a nonvirulent phenotype. A preclinical example of this is seen with administration of a nonantibiotic, high-molecular-weight polymer that protects mice inoculated with typically virulent organisms from mortality by altering their phenotype.[38] A further example of the how the host response is altered by the microbiome can be seen when studying germ free mice, which are raised in microisolator cages and lack an endogenous microflora. When germ-free mice are given *P aeruginosa* pneumonia, they have a significantly higher mortality compared with wild-type mice[39]; however, germ-free mice subjected to hemorrhagic shock or ischemia–reperfusion injuries have an improved survival compared with mice with intact, normal gut microflora.[40,41]

## GUT FAILURE IN CRITICALLY ILL PATIENTS

### *Clinical Diagnosis of Gut Failure*

Symptoms of gut failure in the ICU are nonspecific and are not included currently in severity scoring symptoms such as the Sequential Organ Failure Assessment score. A recent prospective multicenter study of 377 patients in the ICU requiring mechanical ventilation sought to determine whether 6 gastroenterological symptoms, namely, high gastric residual volumes, absent bowel sounds, vomiting/regurgitation, diarrhea, bowel distension, and gastrointestinal bleeding, could predict patient outcome.[42] None of the symptoms[43] alone was an independent predictor of mortality. However, when 3 or more symptoms were present at day 1 of ICU stay, there was a 3-fold increase in the risk of mortality.

Additionally, analysis of patient stool samples has shown promise in predicting outcomes. In a study of nearly 500 stool samples from an ICU cohort with sepsis, it was determined that when fecal pH goes up or down by 1, the incidence of bacteremia more than triples and mortality more than doubles.[44] Further, a decrease in obligate and facultative anaerobes has been shown to correlate with increased risk of mortality in patients with the systemic inflammatory response syndrome, whereas a depleted or single pattern fecal stain for bacteria is associated with a greater risk of mortality in MODS compared with a diverse pattern.[43]

Although not commonly used clinically, biomarkers have shown significant promise in diagnosing gut failure. The concentration of plasma citrulline is a marker of enterocyte functional metabolic mass, so decreased serum citrulline is a potential marker of intestinal damage. Further, intestinal fatty acid-binding protein is localized in enterocytes and is released after enterocyte damage, so an increase in this protein is also a potential marker of intestinal damage. The importance of both citrulline and intestinal fatty acid binding protein was recently shown in a series of more than 100 medical intensive care unit patients, of which 15% had septic shock and 20% had acute respiratory distress syndrome.[45] Increased intestinal fatty acid binding protein on ICU admission was associated with catecholamine support, higher lactate, higher Sequential Organ Failure Assessment score, and higher International Normalized Ratio, whereas decreased citrulline was associated with higher intraabdominal pressure, greater C-reactive protein concentration, and more frequent antibiotic use. Alterations in both were associated with greater 28-day mortality. Of note, 2 additional studies found increased serum intestinal fatty acid binding protein in patients with acute mesenteric ischemia.[46,47]

## TARGETING THE MICROBIOME

Clinical strategies aimed at augmenting, decreasing, or transplanting the microbiome are all used in clinical practice to varying degrees. Despite the widely varying intellectual basis for each of these as a potential therapeutic, each has shown some potential benefit, although their efficacy and potential unwanted side effects remain incompletely understood.

### *Probiotics, Prebiotics, and Synbiotics*

Because microbial diversity has been shown to be associated with outcomes in critical illness, the concept of augmenting "good" bacteria and restoring microbial ecology is potentially beneficial with the goal of restoring a normal, diverse flora. This can be done in a number of complementary ways: (a) probiotics are exogenous live organisms, (b) prebiotics are nondigestible nutrients that stimulate commensal bacterial growth, and (c) synbiotics are a combination of probiotics and prebiotics. The theoretic benefit of each of these is multifactorial, including local release of antimicrobial factors, maintenance of gut barrier integrity, competition for epithelial adherence, prevention of bacterial translocation, and modulation of the local immune response.[48] Two recent meta-analyses of probiotics in more than 1000 patients in the ICU demonstrate a decrease in the incidence of ventilator-associated pneumonia, with one showing a decreased length of stay.[49,50] No alteration in mortality was noted. It should be noted that the largest trial of probiotics to date showed increased mortality (16% vs 6%) in 296 patients with severe pancreatitis.[51] However, this trial has been heavily criticized,[52] and does not seem to be representative of other studies of probiotics. Multiple questions remain before augmenting the microbiome gaining widespread usage as a strategy to improve outcomes in the ICU. These include what (if any) the optimal probiotic agent is, if combinations of agents are more beneficial, if synbiotics are superior to probiotics alone, what the ideal "dose", is and what the long-term safety profile is.

### *Selective Decontamination of the Digestive Tract*

In contrast with augmenting the microbiome, selective decontamination of the digestive tract (SDD) seeks to preferentially minimize pathogenic enteral bacteria. The goal of this practice is to eradicate oropharyngeal and intestinal carriage of pathogenic microorganisms without adversely impacting the remaining microbiome on either the patient level or the ICU level. SDD includes 3 components: (a) 4 to 5 days of parenteral antibiotics (cefotaxime in previously healthy patients, combination therapy or antipseudomonal cephalosporin in patients with chronic disease), (b) nonabsorbable enteral antibiotics given via nasoenteric tube given throughout the ICU stay, and (c) pastes or gels applied to the oropharynx.[53] It should be noted that the term "selective" is a bit of a misnomer, because this approach targets both normal and abnormal flora, and does not cover multiple low-level pathogens.

For a practice that is used rarely worldwide (with certain exceptions), the data on SDD are both robust and impressive. In fact, it is a great paradox that the sheer volume of studies on this practice might be greater (and more supportive) than in almost any aspect of critical care, yet this has not translated to a change in clinical practice. Specifically, there have been more than 60 randomized controlled trials and more than 10 metaanalyses on SDD in more than 15,000 patients, demonstrating a reduction of lower airway infection of 72% and bloodstream infection by 37%.[54,55]

Given this significant literature, why is SDD not used more commonly used? The answer relates exclusively to concerns related to the development of antibiotic resistance. Although the majority of studies examining this issue have not demonstrated the development of resistance (although a few have), these have generally been performed in ICUs that have low levels of antibiotic resistance at baseline.[56] With increasing attention being paid to antibiotic stewardship and resistance worldwide, the fear that widespread antibiotic usage for preventive purposes will induce new and difficult or impossible to treat "superbugs" has limited adoption of SDD. Further, with an increased understanding of the importance of microbial health and diversity, it is currently unclear how these are impacted by the use of SDD in critically ill patients.

### *Fecal Transplant*

There has recently been an explosion of interest in fecal microbiota transplant, where stool from a healthy donor is given to a recipient with the goal of restoring the microbiome to its homeostatic state seen in health. Although multiple indications are currently being studied, the most convincing data are in recurrent *Clostridium difficile* infection, where cure rates are 3 times higher than seen with conventional medical therapy without apparent side effects.[57] To date, fecal transplant is not typically used in critically ill patients because antibiotic use (which is common in the ICU) would immediately change the microbial components of a patient's stool (either from donor or recipient) after the transplant.

### *Nutrition*

Although a comprehensive review of nutritional support is outside the scope of this review, it is worth emphasizing the importance of nutritional support in the ICU, as one of the major roles of the healthy intestine is to absorb nutrients. Enteral nutrition is preferable to parenteral nutrition because enteral nutrition has beneficial effects on gut-associated lymphoid tissue and mucosal health, and not does have the increased risk of infection associated with parenteral nutrition. Enteral nutrition should be initiated within 48 hours of ICU admission if possible.

## REFERENCES

1. Mittal R, Coopersmith CM. Redefining the gut as the motor of critical illness. Trends Mol Med 2014;20(4):214–23.
2. Clark JA, Coopersmith CM. Intestinal crosstalk: a new paradigm for understanding the gut as the "motor" of critical illness. Shock 2007;28(4):384–93.
3. Carrico CJ, Meakins JL, Marshall JC, et al. Multiple-organ-failure syndrome. The gastrointestinal tract: the "motor" of MOF. Arch Surg 1986;121(2):196–208.
4. Helander HF, Fandriks L. Surface area of the digestive tract - revisited. Scand J Gastroenterol 2014;49(6):681–9.
5. Clevers HC, Bevins CL. Paneth cells: maestros of the small intestinal crypts. Annu Rev Physiol 2013;75:289–311.
6. Galperin C, Gershwin ME. Immunopathogenesis of gastrointestinal and hepatobiliary diseases. JAMA 1997;278(22):1946–55.
7. Schulz O, Pabst O. Antigen sampling in the small intestine. Trends Immunol 2013; 34(4):155–61.
8. Defazio J, Fleming ID, Shakhsheer B, et al. The opposing forces of the intestinal microbiome and the emerging pathobiome. Surg Clin North Am 2014;94(6): 1151–61.
9. Xu Z, Knight R. Dietary effects on human gut microbiome diversity. Br J Nutr 2015;113(Suppl):S1–5.
10. Earley ZM, Akhtar S, Green SJ, et al. Burn injury alters the intestinal microbiome and increases gut permeability and bacterial translocation. PLoS One 2015; 10(7):e0129996.
11. Moore FA, Moore EE, Poggetti R, et al. Gut bacterial translocation via the portal vein: a clinical perspective with major torso trauma. J Trauma 1991;31(5):629–36.
12. Purohit V, Bode JC, Bode C, et al. Alcohol, intestinal bacterial growth, intestinal permeability to endotoxin, and medical consequences: summary of a symposium. Alcohol 2008;42(5):349–61.
13. Badami CD, Senthil M, Caputo FJ, et al. Mesenteric lymph duct ligation improves survival in a lethal shock model. Shock 2008;30(6):680–5.
14. Deitch EA. Gut-origin sepsis: evolution of a concept. Surgeon 2012;10(6):350–6.
15. Senthil M, Watkins A, Barlos D, et al. Intravenous injection of trauma-hemorrhagic shock mesenteric lymph causes lung injury that is dependent upon activation of the inducible nitric oxide synthase pathway. Ann Surg 2007;246(5):822–30.
16. Dominguez JA, Xie Y, Dunne WM, et al. Intestine-specific Mttp deletion decreases mortality and prevents sepsis-induced intestinal injury in a murine model of Pseudomonas aeruginosa pneumonia. PLoS One 2012;7(11):e49159.

17. Liang Z, Xie Y, Dominguez JA, et al. Intestine-specific deletion of microsomal triglyceride transfer protein increases mortality in aged mice. PLoS One 2014;9(7): e101828.
18. Hiramatsu M, Hotchkiss RS, Karl IE, et al. Cecal ligation and puncture (CLP) induces apoptosis in thymus, spleen, lung, and gut by an endotoxin and TNF-independent pathway. Shock 1997;7(4):247–53.
19. Hotchkiss RS, Swanson PE, Freeman BD, et al. Apoptotic cell death in patients with sepsis, shock, and multiple organ dysfunction. Crit Care Med 1999;27(7): 1230–51.
20. Coopersmith CM, Stromberg PE, Dunne WM, et al. Inhibition of intestinal epithelial apoptosis and survival in a murine model of pneumonia-induced sepsis. JAMA 2002;287(13):1716–21.
21. Coopersmith CM, Chang KC, Swanson PE, et al. Overexpression of Bcl-2 in the intestinal epithelium improves survival in septic mice. Crit Care Med 2002;30(1): 195–201.
22. Fox AC, Breed ER, Liang Z, et al. Prevention of lymphocyte apoptosis in septic mice with cancer increases mortality. J Immunol 2011;187(4):1950–6.
23. Stromberg PE, Woolsey CA, Clark AT, et al. CD4+ lymphocytes control gut epithelial apoptosis and mediate survival in sepsis. FASEB J 2009;23(6): 1817–25.
24. Iwata A, Stevenson VM, Minard A, et al. Over-expression of Bcl-2 provides protection in septic mice by a trans effect. J Immunol 2003;171(6):3136–41.
25. Bischoff SC, Barbara G, Buurman W, et al. Intestinal permeability–a new target for disease prevention and therapy. BMC Gastroenterol 2014;14:189.
26. Cunningham KE, Turner JR. Myosin light chain kinase: pulling the strings of epithelial tight junction function. Ann N Y Acad Sci 2012;1258:34–42.
27. Odenwald MA, Turner JR. Intestinal permeability defects: is it time to treat? Clin Gastroenterol Hepatol 2013;11(9):1075–83.
28. Fink MP. Intestinal epithelial hyperpermeability: update on the pathogenesis of gut mucosal barrier dysfunction in critical illness. Curr Opin Crit Care 2003; 9(2):143–51.
29. Fredenburgh LE, Velandia MM, Ma J, et al. Cyclooxygenase-2 deficiency leads to intestinal barrier dysfunction and increased mortality during polymicrobial sepsis. J Immunol 2011;187(10):5255–67.
30. Chen C, Wang P, Su Q, et al. Myosin light chain kinase mediates intestinal barrier disruption following burn injury. PLoS ONE 2012;7(4):e34946.
31. Zahs A, Bird MD, Ramirez L, et al. Inhibition of long myosin light-chain kinase activation alleviates intestinal damage after binge ethanol exposure and burn injury. Am J Physiol Gastrointest Liver Physiol 2012;303(6):G705–12.
32. Clark JA, Clark AT, Hotchkiss RS, et al. Epidermal growth factor treatment decreases mortality and is associated with improved gut integrity in sepsis. Shock 2008;30(1):36–42.
33. Dominguez JA, Vithayathil PJ, Khailova L, et al. Epidermal growth factor improves survival and prevents intestinal injury in a murine model of pseudomonas aeruginosa pneumonia. Shock 2011;36(4):381–9.
34. Clark JA, Gan H, Samocha AJ, et al. Enterocyte-specific epidermal growth factor prevents barrier dysfunction and improves mortality in murine peritonitis. Am J Physiol Gastrointest Liver Physiol 2009;297(3):G471–9.
35. Babrowski T, Romanowski K, Fink D, et al. The intestinal environment of surgical injury transforms Pseudomonas aeruginosa into a discrete hypervirulent morphotype capable of causing lethal peritonitis. Surgery 2013;153(1):36–43.

36. Zaborina O, Lepine F, Xiao G, et al. Dynorphin activates quorum sensing quinolone signaling in pseudomonas aeruginosa. PLoS Pathog 2007;3(3):e35.
37. Wu L, Estrada O, Zaborina O, et al. Recognition of host immune activation by Pseudomonas aeruginosa. Science 2005;309(5735):774–7.
38. Zaborin A, Defazio JR, Kade M, et al. Phosphate-containing polyethylene glycol polymers prevent lethal sepsis by multidrug-resistant pathogens. Antimicrob Agents Chemother 2014;58(2):966–77.
39. Fox AC, McConnell KW, Yoseph BP, et al. The endogenous bacteria alter gut epithelial apoptosis and decrease mortality following Pseudomonas aeruginosa pneumonia. Shock 2012;38(5):508–14.
40. Ferraro FJ, Rush BF Jr, Simonian GT, et al. A comparison of survival at different degrees of hemorrhagic shock in germ-free and germ-bearing rats. Shock 1995;4(2):117–20.
41. Fagundes CT, Amaral FA, Vieira AT, et al. Transient TLR activation restores inflammatory response and ability to control pulmonary bacterial infection in germfree mice. J Immunol 2012;188(3):1411–20.
42. Reintam BA, Poeze M, Malbrain ML, et al. Gastrointestinal symptoms during the first week of intensive care are associated with poor outcome: a prospective multicentre study. Intensive Care Med 2013;39(5):899–909.
43. Shimizu K, Ogura H, Hamasaki T, et al. Altered gut flora are associated with septic complications and death in critically ill patients with systemic inflammatory response syndrome. Dig Dis Sci 2011;56(4):1171–7.
44. Osuka A, Shimizu K, Ogura H, et al. Prognostic impact of fecal pH in critically ill patients. Crit Care 2012;16(4):R119.
45. Piton G, Belon F, Cypriani B, et al. Enterocyte damage in critically ill patients is associated with shock condition and 28-day mortality. Crit Care Med 2013;41(9):2169–76.
46. Thuijls G, van WK, Grootjans J, et al. Early diagnosis of intestinal ischemia using urinary and plasma fatty acid binding proteins. Ann Surg 2011;253(2):303–8.
47. Guzel M, Sozuer EM, Salt O, et al. Value of the serum I-FABP level for diagnosing acute mesenteric ischemia. Surg Today 2014;44(11):2072–6.
48. Theodorakopoulou M, Perros E, Giamarellos-Bourboulis EJ, et al. Controversies in the management of the critically ill: the role of probiotics. Int J Antimicrob Agents 2013;42(Suppl):S41–4.
49. Bo L, Li J, Tao T, et al. Probiotics for preventing ventilator-associated pneumonia. Cochrane Database Syst Rev 2014;(10):CD009066.
50. Barraud D, Bollaert PE, Gibot S. Impact of the administration of probiotics on mortality in critically ill adult patients: a meta-analysis of randomized controlled trials. Chest 2013;143(3):646–55.
51. Besselink MG, van Santvoort HC, Buskens E, et al. Probiotic prophylaxis in predicted severe acute pancreatitis: a randomised, double-blind, placebo-controlled trial. Lancet 2008;371(9613):651–9.
52. Expression of concern–Probiotic prophylaxis in predicted severe acute pancreatitis: a randomised, double-blind, placebo-controlled trial. Lancet 2010;375(9718):875–6.
53. Silvestri L, van Saene HK. Selective decontamination of the digestive tract: an update of the evidence. HSR Proc Intensive Care Cardiovasc Anesth 2012;4(1):21–9.
54. Petros AJ, Silvestri L, van Saene HK, et al. 2B or not 2B for selective decontamination of the digestive tract in the surviving sepsis campaign guidelines. Crit Care Med 2013;41(11):e385–6.

55. Silvestri L, de La Cal MA, van Saene HK. Selective decontamination of the digestive tract: the mechanism of action is control of gut overgrowth. Intensive Care Med 2012;38(11):1738–50.
56. de Smet AM, Kluytmans JA, Blok HE, et al. Selective digestive tract decontamination and selective oropharyngeal decontamination and antibiotic resistance in patients in intensive-care units: an open-label, clustered group-randomised, crossover study. Lancet Infect Dis 2011;11(5):372–80.
57. Drekonja D, Reich J, Gezahegn S, et al. Fecal microbiota transplantation for Clostridium difficile infection: a systematic review. Ann Intern Med 2015;162(9):630–8.

# Abdominal Compartment Hypertension and Abdominal Compartment Syndrome

Patrick Maluso, MD[a], Jody Olson, MD[b,c], Babak Sarani, MD[d,*]

**KEYWORDS**

• Abdominal compartment syndrome • Abdominal hypertension

**KEY POINTS**

- Abdominal compartment hypertension and syndrome should be expected following resuscitation in patients with an increase in the intraperitoneal contents (including tense ascites), and in those with decreased abdominal wall compliance.
- Measurement of bladder pressure is the standard of care by which intra-abdominal pressure should be measured in the intensive care unit in most instances.
- Abdominal hypertension is present when abdominal pressure exceeds 12 mm Hg and abdominal compartment syndrome is present with abdominal pressure exceeds 25 mm Hg.
- Although decompressive laparotomy is definitive treatment of all cases of abdominal compartment syndrome, some causes, such as tense ascites or hemoperitoneum, can be treated with paracentesis, and decreased abdominal wall compliance can be treated with pharmacologic paralysis and deep sedation.

## INTRODUCTION

Abdominal compartment syndrome (ACS) is a rare but clinically significant outcome in critical illness. Although ACS is the most severe end point on a spectrum of disease related to increased intraperitoneal pressure, it is preceded by intra-abdominal hypertension (IAH), which is less likely to be associated with end-organ dysfunction.

Disclosure: The authors have nothing to disclose.

[a] Department of Surgery, George Washington University, 2150 Pennsylvania Avenue, Northwest, Suite 6B, Washington, DC 20037, USA; [b] Division of Hepatology, University of Kansas, 3901 Rainbow Boulevard, MS 1023, Kansas City, KS 66160, USA; [c] Division of Liver Transplantation, University of Kansas, 3901 Rainbow Boulevard, MS 1023, Kansas City, KS 66160, USA; [d] Department of Surgery, Center for Trauma and Critical Care, George Washington University, 2150 Pennsylvania Avenue, Northwest, Suite 6B, Washington, DC 20037, USA
* Corresponding author.
*E-mail address:* bsarani@mfa.gwu.edu

Crit Care Clin 32 (2016) 213–222
http://dx.doi.org/10.1016/j.ccc.2015.12.001 criticalcare.theclinics.com
0749-0704/16/$ – see front matter 

Although the exact incidence of either condition is poorly defined, the few available reports on the subject show that ACS occurs in between 10% and 35% of noninjured critically ill patients.[1] This rate also mirrors the incidence of ACS following major operation or trauma.[2,3] IAH, which has broader inclusion criteria than ACS, has a higher incidence than might be expected. Although also poorly defined, 30% to 70% of either subset of patients develop IAH. In both medical and surgical critical care patients, the presence of IAH or ACS is associated with a significant increase in mortality.

At the most basic level, IAH and ACS are physiologically similar to compartment syndromes in general and result in a derangement of tissue perfusion caused by increased pressure within the fixed volume of an anatomic compartment. The abdomen and pelvis collectively form one such compartment, bounded by the diaphragm, abdominal wall, back, and the peritoneal reflection at the bony pelvis. As with other compartment syndromes, increased pressures within the fixed abdominal compartment impair capillary and venous blood flow, thereby ultimately decreasing arteriole flow as well. The resultant cellular hypoxia leads to anaerobic respiration and lactic acidosis. This metabolic acidosis is often worsened by a respiratory acidosis arising from upward pressure on the diaphragm that prevents adequate ventilation and $CO_2$ exchange. Other common impairments seen in ACS include malperfusion of the intestines caused by decreased venous outflow from the splanchnic circulation, acute kidney injury caused by decreased glomerular blood flow, and decreased cardiac return as a result of compression of the inferior vena cava. Left unchecked, these events can lead to significant systemic acidosis and cardiovascular collapse.

## DEFINITION AND CAUSES OF INTRA-ABDOMINAL HYPERTENSION/ABDOMINAL COMPARTMENT SYNDROME

The most commonly used definition of ACS was published by the World Society on Abdominal Compartment Syndrome (WSACS) in 2013.[4] This consensus document addresses clinical definitions and pressure measurement guidelines intended to assist clinicians and researchers in the diagnosis, treatment, and characterization of IAH/ACS. Intra-abdominal pressure (IAP) is defined as the end-expiratory abdominal pressure in the supine position in the setting of fully relaxed abdominal wall musculature. Measured IAP is used to calculate the abdominal perfusion pressure (APP) by subtracting IAP from the systemic mean arterial pressure (MAP); in this sense, APP can be thought of as the abdominal analog to cerebral perfusion pressure and can be used as a predictor of visceral perfusion. The WSACS statement defines IAH as a sustained IAP greater than 12 mm Hg, in contrast with normal IAP, which ranges from 2 to 7 mm Hg. IAH is further subdivided into grades I to IV (**Table 1**).

**Table 1**
**Grading and treatment of IAH**

| Grade | IAP (mm Hg) | Treatments |
|---|---|---|
| I | 12–15 | Sedate patient, diurese, paracentesis, loosen abdominal closure device |
| II | 16–20 | Sedate patient, diurese, paracentesis, loosen abdominal closure device |
| III | 21–25 | Pharmacologically paralyze patient, loosen abdominal closure device, decompressive laparotomy |
| IV | >25 | Decompressive laparotomy |

ACS is defined as IAH with sustained IAP greater than 20 mm Hg (IAH grades III and IV) with or without an APP less than 60 mm Hg and is accompanied by end-organ dysfunction. Confounding factors such as obesity can affect patients' baseline IAP and therefore should be considered when assessing patients for IAH, although there are no guidelines as to how to account for obesity-associated IAH quantitatively. Sanchez and colleagues[5] published a prospective study of IAP in morbidly obese patients and showed a strong correlation between body mass index (BMI) and IAP. Wilson and colleagues[6] studied IAP in anesthetized bariatric surgical patients and found that baseline IAP increased by 0.14 mm Hg for every unit of BMI; however, none of the patients' baseline IAPs were pathologic. The mean baseline IAP measured in the cohort was 9 ± 6 mm Hg with an average BMI of 48 kg/m$^2$.

There are many patient, illnesses, and therapeutic intervention risk factors related to the development of IAH; however, it is difficult to predict which patients will ultimately develop IAH. In general, IAH can result from decreased abdominal wall compliance, an increase in the volume of abdominal contents, or a combination of the two. Impaired abdominal wall compliance is commonly altered in the setting of burns, abdominal wall operations (especially ventral herniorrhaphy), and prone positioning.[6,7] Large-volume fluid resuscitation can increase intra-abdominal volume indirectly by causing bowel edema as well as directly by creating ascites, and is common in patients with sepsis, trauma, and burns.[4,8,9] The volume of intra-abdominal contents can be directly increased by space-occupying lesions such as large tumors, tense ascites, hemoperitoneum, severe ileus, and pancreatitis, all of which have also been implicated in the development of IAH.[4,8,10] In addition, patients with a history of ascites caused by advanced liver disease and/or portal hypertension are at risk for IAH and ACS when critically ill. Because it is difficult to predict who will develop IAH and ACS, it is important to understand the underlying pathophysiology that predisposes patients to IAH and have a heightened clinical index of suspicion to identify patients with risk factors for the disorder.

Large-volume crystalloid-based resuscitation is strongly associated with development of both IAH and ACS.[9] The incidence of ACS decreases significantly when a colloid, particularly blood and plasma, or hypertonic-based resuscitation strategy is used in lieu of large-volume, crystalloid-based strategy.[11,12]

## DIAGNOSIS: PHYSIOLOGIC MARKERS OF ABDOMINAL COMPARTMENT SYNDROME

Early recognition of IAH is the essential first step in preventing ACS. A protocol for initiation of IAP measurements based on known risk factors and/or clinical suspicion is vital. IAP should be measured in patients with 2 or more of the risk factors listed in **Box 1**.[13]

Cephalad pressure on the diaphragm decreases functional residual capacity and tidal volume.[14] This degradation in lung volumes is exacerbated by increasing IAP.[15] Patients with ACS require mechanical ventilation because of an inability to adequately ventilate spontaneously. The use of mechanical ventilation also provides another modality for the recognition of IAH, namely through increased peak inspiratory, plateau, and mean airway pressures.[16] The hypoventilation resultant from decreased pulmonary compliance initially manifests as hypercapnic respiratory failure but can progress to hypoxemia.[17,18]

IAH and ACS have multiple hemodynamic sequelae. Both result in decreased venous return to the heart caused by compression of the inferior vena cava and transmitted increases in intrathoracic pressure (ITP). This effect is magnified by hypovolemia. In addition to decreasing venous return, increased ITP also decreases cardiac

**Box 1**
**Risk factors for IAH**

- High-volume fluid resuscitation
  - Septic shock
  - Hemorrhagic shock, particularly when resuscitated using crystalloid solutions in lieu of colloid/blood products
  - Large-surface-area burn
  - Pancreatitis
- Decreased abdominal wall compliance
  - Large or circumferential torso burn
  - Ventral hernia repair with tight abdominal wall closure
  - Prone positioning
- Increased abdominal content
  - Tense ascites in patients with cirrhosis
  - Large neoplasm
  - Pancreatitis

filling by decreasing right ventricular compliance.[17,18] At very increased levels, high IAP can also increase systemic vascular resistance by compressing the aorta and splanchnic circulation, resulting in increased afterload and reduced stroke volume.[17,18] Ultimately, patients experience a net decrease in cardiac output with resultant hypotension.[19]

Renal dysfunction is also common in ACS and manifests as oliguria when IAP is greater than 15 mm Hg or anuria when IAP exceeds 30 mm Hg. Acute kidney injury in ACS is caused by both prerenal and tubular processes. In a canine model, IAP of 20 mm Hg or more increased renal vascular resistance by 555%.[20] The decreased cardiac output described earlier contributes to prerenal failure; however, IAH is also an independent cause of renal impairment.[21] IAH reduces renal plasma flow and glomerular filtration rate through compression of the renal arteriole and venous circulation and of the tubules themselves.[22] Taken together, this compression leads to increased activation of the renin-angiotensin-aldosterone hormone signaling cascade and thereby increases systemic vascular resistance. This process ultimately leads to further worsening of the cardiac output, as described earlier.[23]

The hepatobiliary system is especially sensitive to the effects of increased IAP, an effect that is independent of derangements in cardiac output. Hepatic venous, arterial, and microcirculatory blood flow decreases significantly with even slight increases in IAP.[24] Hepatic impairment manifests through impaired clearance of plasma lactate, resulting in metabolic acidosis that is not solely attributable to increased production of lactate.[25] This deficient clearance can confuse the clinical interpretation of lactate levels, rendering them less reliable in their common use as a resuscitative end point when measured in patients with IAH. Moreover, increases in serum lactate levels depress the serum pH, which can result in decreased myocardial contractility. Lactic acidosis can also cause systemic arteriolar dilation, which further depresses the systemic blood pressure, impairs cellular respiration, and further increases lactic acid production, effectively creating a feedback loop that accelerates physiologic deterioration.

The effects of increased IAP on bowel perfusion also worsen the lactic acidosis seen in IAH. In a porcine model, IAP of 20 mm Hg has been shown to impair mesenteric circulation with a resultant decrease in mucosal blood flow and in measured mucosal pH.[24] Other studies have shown inadequate intestinal mucosal oxygen levels in the setting of IAH, further supporting the notion of bowel ischemia caused by increased IAP.[26] Intestinal ischemia can manifest as interstitial edema and/or ileus, both of which increase intra-abdominal volume and worsen ACS.

Bowel ischemia predisposes patients to further physiologic decompensation by a mechanism independent of those described in previous sections. After 60 minutes of sustained IAP of more than 25 mm Hg, mucosal blood flow is impaired even in well-resuscitated patients (as shown by normal MAPs), and has been shown to allow translocation of intraluminal bacteria across the damaged mucosal barrier.[27] This bacterial translocation can result in sepsis or septic shock if ACS is not recognized and treated expeditiously, further contributing to the numerous aforementioned physiologic derangements that may result in the rapid clinical deterioration or death of the patient.

## DIAGNOSIS: MEASUREMENT OF ABDOMINAL PRESSURE

Clinical examination alone is insufficient in the diagnosis of IAH. In a prospective study of 110 consecutive intensive care unit (ICU) patients who had undergone abdominal surgery, an intensivist's clinical estimation of IAP was compared with a quantified measurement and was shown to have only 61% sensitivity for detecting an IAP greater than 18 mm Hg.[2,28] Because clinical examination alone is unreliable, objective IAP measurements are necessary to guide management of critically ill patients with suspected IAH or ACS. Multiple direct and indirect methods for measurement of IAP have been described.

Measuring IAP directly is theoretically the most accurate method but requires access to the peritoneal compartment, exposing patients to the risks associated with invasive abdominal procedures. These techniques are therefore not broadly useful in screening for IAH. Direct measurement of IAP can be achieved by placement of intraperitoneal pressure transducers. However, introduction of such a catheter exposes patients to unnecessary risk of complications unless there are indications for drainage of ascites that outweigh the risk associated with violation of the peritoneum. Because of this, direct measurements are usually only obtained through measurement of pressures across extant peritoneal dialysis catheters or indwelling ascites drainage catheters used for palliation of malignant ascites.

Indirect measurement techniques are numerous and common. As described earlier, the ventilator may allow measurement of peak ventilator pressures, although alterations in lung and chest wall compliance from other processes also contribute to increased peak pressures and can limit the utility of the ventilator in diagnosis of IAH. Other indirect measurement methods use central venous, intravesical, rectal, and intrauterine pressures to assess IAP. However, each has unique strengths and limitations. Measurement of intravesical pressure is generally considered the gold standard among indirect methods for diagnosis of IAH because of its ease and minimally invasive nature.[4,13] This technique should be performed in fully supine patients to remove the confounding effects of patient position on IAP. In keeping with the WSACS definition of IAH, IAP is measured at end-expiration with the abdominal wall musculature fully relaxed. Ideally, this necessitates use of deep chemical sedation and pharmacologic paralysis, although the pressure is frequently measured without paralysis. Intravesical pressure is measured by instillation of 20 mL of sterile water or saline into the bladder via a urinary catheter attached to a manometer zeroed at the level of the midaxillary line. This standardized technique allows measurement of the pressure that is transmitted from the abdomen. The procedure must be performed with proper sterile technique using sterile fluids in order to prevent iatrogenic urinary tract infections. Instillation of more than 50 mL into the catheter artificially increases the measured IAP, as shown in a prospective trial of serial IAP measurements with intravesical manometry.[29] There are commercially available products that connect to urinary catheters and, through standardization of materials and methods, may decrease the probability of technical error when measuring abdominal pressure. However, these systems may be cost-prohibitive or simply unavailable in certain clinical settings. A needle introduced into the sampling port of a standard urinary catheter and connected to a pressure transducer can provide an alternative means of measurement.

Although intravesical manometry is the gold standard for indirect measurement of IAP, it is impossible, contraindicated, or may not be accurate in those with a history of cystectomy, traumatic bladder injury, or pelvic packing, respectively. In these patient cohorts, a variety of other measurement techniques may be substituted for intravesical manometry. Several investigators have suggested the use of a standard central venous catheter to measure inferior vena caval pressures. Inferior vena caval pressure measurements have shown good correlation with pressures obtained through other validated methods.[30] Intragastric pressures are another alternative means of indirectly measuring IAP and are obtained using nasogastric or orogastric tube manometry; however, intermittent measurements obtained with this technique can be unreliable because of the confounding effects of increased pressure caused by gastric contractions. Continuous pressure monitoring using an intragastric balloon may be useful in overcoming this limitation and has been validated by comparison with direct measurement of IAP following abdominal insufflation to a known pressure during laparoscopic cholecystectomy.[31] Although this technique overcomes the confounding effects of gastric contractions, other factors, such as the administration of enteral feeds, may confound the measurements; an effect that is insufficiently characterized in the literature. Other novel techniques using specialized catheters with embedded microchips to measure intravesical, rectal, or intrauterine pressures have been described but are less cost-effective than the simpler techniques described earlier and are not widely available.[32]

Most studies use absolute IAP in their analyses, but a recent retrospective study found that APP may be a more clinically useful end point in the diagnosis and treatment of IAH. Cheatham and colleagues[33] conducted a retrospective review of 144 patients treated for IAH. APP was a better predictor of mortality compared with other commonly used clinical end points such as serum lactate level or urine output. Furthermore, an APP of less than 60 mm Hg reliably predicted the need for urgent intervention, demonstrating the usefulness of APP as both a resuscitative goal and as a predictor of need for definitive surgical decompression. In another study, Al-Dorzi and colleagues[28] conducted a post-hoc analysis of a double-blind, randomized, placebo-controlled trial involving cirrhotic patients with septic shock. Lower initial APP was associated with increased mortality. Although the WSACS defines normal APP as greater than 60 mm Hg, this study found a breakpoint of APP less than or equal to 55 mm Hg as a predictor of survival and found that this measurement was superior to traditional resuscitative end points, such as MAP or central venous oxygen saturation, in predicting mortality, leading the investigators to suggest its use as a resuscitative end point for cirrhotics with septic shock. The WSACS makes no recommendation regarding the use of APP as a resuscitative end point[13]; however, the limited data on its use are promising. Further study is needed in broader patient populations to determine the clinical relevance of APP in critically ill patients.

## TREATMENT

Appropriate treatment of ACS requires rapid normalization of the IAP, thereby restoring normal abdominal visceral perfusion and resolving the aforementioned cardiopulmonary functional impairments. Definitive management of ACS from most causes other than tense ascites, which can be treated by large-volume paracentesis, involves emergent surgical decompression of the abdomen via a midline laparotomy, often performed at the bedside in the ICU. However, this may be extremely morbid and should be reserved for only the most severe forms of IAH or true ACS. Lower-grade IAH may be temporized or relieved using nonsurgical measures (see **Table 1**). Increased abdominal wall tension caused by burns, third-spacing of fluids into the abdominal wall, or a tight abdominal wall repair following ventral herniorrhaphy can create a lower-grade IAH that may be improved through the use of neuromuscular blockade (NMB) to reduce IAP. A prospective study of patients with IAH showed an average reduction of IAP of 4 mm Hg after administration of cisatracurium; however, the response was short-lived. Moreover, the use of NMB did not increase patients' APPs, suggesting that NMB has limited clinical utility in the definitive treatment of IAH and that it is ineffective for management of true ACS.[34] Nevertheless, NMB may be useful as a temporizing measure when definitive surgical management is not readily available or feasible.

In patients with IAH caused by acutely increased intraperitoneal volumes, as seen in large-volume crystalloid infusion or tense ascites, paracentesis is effective in avoiding the morbidity associated with decompressive laparotomy.[35] Similarly, paracentesis has a demonstrated efficacy in the relief of IAH caused by massive ascites in cirrhotic patients. Savino and colleagues[36] showed improvement in cardiac index, urinary output, and creatinine clearance after drainage of sufficient ascitic fluid to reduce the IAP by 10 mm Hg. These results suggest that percutaneous drainage of free intraperitoneal fluid may have at least a temporizing role, if not a definitive one, in the management of IAH resulting from large volumes of peritoneal fluid. When large-volume paracentesis is performed in cirrhotic patients, attention to prevention and treatment of postparacentesis circulatory dysfunction is imperative. Strategies include 20% to 25% albumin replacement at a dose of 8 g per liter of ascites removed and/or treatment with vasopressor agents to maintain an appropriate mean arterial and renal perfusion pressure.[37,38]

All of the aforementioned therapeutic modalities have limited roles in the temporization and management of IAH and should therefore be attempted where clinically indicated. Nevertheless, patients with ACS have organ system dysfunction by definition and therefore require emergent definitive management with decompressive laparotomy in most cases.[13,29] However, laparotomy inherently confers significant morbidity, and patients' overall clinical presentation should be carefully considered before the decision is made to proceed with surgical decompression of the abdomen. The appropriate setting for the operation should be determined after consideration of the patient's fitness for transport to an operating room. Other important considerations when determining the most appropriate setting for laparotomy include the acuity of patient presentation and level of response to temporizing measures, assessment of the need for high-level positive pressure ventilation that may not be amenable to transport without a ventilator, the availability of adequate portable ventilators, availability and level of training of ancillary and surgical staff, and the ready availability of surgical equipment within the ICU. Moreover, these considerations should be balanced with the risk of ICU laparotomy given that hemorrhage control and maintenance of a sterile environment are significantly more difficult outside the operating room.

## SUMMARY

The resuscitation of critically ill or injured patients can result in IAH and ACS. In addition, certain chronic medical conditions, such as cirrhosis, portend significant risk for

IAH and ACS when patients are critically ill. There is a significant morbidity and mortality risk associated with a delay in recognition and treatment of these conditions. Early diagnosis is the key first step in mitigating these risks; however, physical examination does not offer a sensitive means to diagnose either disorder, necessitating routine monitoring of IAP in patients at risk for IAH or ACS. When significantly increased pressures are detected, clinicians should perform urgent interventions to decrease the IAP.

## REFERENCES


1. Vidal MG, Ruiz Weisser J, Gonzalez F, et al. Incidence and clinical effects of intra-abdominal hypertension in critically ill patients. Crit Care Med 2008;36:1823–31.
2. Balogh Z, McKinley BA, Cocanour CS, et al. Secondary abdominal compartment syndrome is an elusive early complication of traumatic shock resuscitation. Am J Surg 2002;184:538–43 [discussion: 543–4].
3. Balogh Z, McKinley BA, Holcomb JB, et al. Both primary and secondary abdominal compartment syndrome can be predicted early and are harbingers of multiple organ failure. J Trauma 2003;54:848–59 [discussion: 859–61].
4. Kirkpatrick AW, Roberts DJ, De Waele J, et al. Intra-abdominal hypertension and the abdominal compartment syndrome: updated consensus definitions and clinical practice guidelines from the World Society of the Abdominal Compartment Syndrome. Intensive Care Med 2013;39:1190–206.
5. Sanchez NC, Tenofsky PL, Dort JM, et al. What is normal intra-abdominal pressure? Am Surg 2001;67:243–8.
6. Wilson A, Longhi J, Goldman C, et al. Intra-abdominal pressure and the morbidly obese patients: the effect of body mass index. J Trauma 2010;69:78–83.
7. Hering R, Wrigge H, Vorwerk R, et al. The effects of prone positioning on intraabdominal pressure and cardiovascular and renal function in patients with acute lung injury. Anesth Analg 2001;92:1226–31.
8. Reintam Blaser A, Parm P, Kitus R, et al. Intra-abdominal hypertension and gastrointestinal symptoms in mechanically ventilated patients. Crit Care Res Pract 2011;2011:982507.
9. Kasotakis G, Duggan M, Li Y, et al. Optimal pressure of abdominal gas insufflation for bleeding control in a severe swine splenic injury model. J Surg Res 2013; 184:931–6.
10. Reintam Blaser A, Parm P, Kitus R, et al. Risk factors for intra-abdominal hypertension in mechanically ventilated patients. Acta Anaesthesiol Scand 2011;55: 607–14.
11. Neal MD, Hoffman MK, Cuschieri J, et al. Crystalloid to packed red blood cell transfusion ratio in the massively transfused patient: when a little goes a long way. J Trauma Acute Care Surg 2012;72:892–8.
12. Holodinsky JK, Roberts DJ, Ball CG, et al. Risk factors for intra-abdominal hypertension and abdominal compartment syndrome among adult intensive care unit patients: a systematic review and meta-analysis. Crit Care 2013;17:R249.
13. Cheatham ML, Malbrain ML, Kirkpatrick A, et al. Results from the International Conference of Experts on intra-abdominal hypertension and abdominal compartment syndrome. II. Recommendations. Intensive Care Med 2007;33:951–62.
14. Obeid F, Saba A, Fath J, et al. Increases in intra-abdominal pressure affect pulmonary compliance. Arch Surg 1995;130:544–7 [discussion: 7–8].
15. Pelosi P, Quintel M, Malbrain ML. Effect of intra-abdominal pressure on respiratory mechanics. Acta Clin Belg 2007;62(Suppl 1):78–88.

16. Gattinoni L, Pelosi P, Suter PM, et al. Acute respiratory distress syndrome caused by pulmonary and extrapulmonary disease. Different syndromes? Am J Respir Crit Care Med 1998;158:3–11.
17. Cullen DJ, Coyle JP, Teplick R, et al. Cardiovascular, pulmonary, and renal effects of massively increased intra-abdominal pressure in critically ill patients. Crit Care Med 1989;17:118–21.
18. Ridings PC, Bloomfield GL, Blocher CR, et al. Cardiopulmonary effects of raised intra-abdominal pressure before and after intravascular volume expansion. J Trauma 1995;39:1071–5.
19. Barnes GE, Laine GA, Giam PY, et al. Cardiovascular responses to elevation of intra-abdominal hydrostatic pressure. Am J Physiol 1985;248:R208–13.
20. Harman PK, Kron IL, McLachlan HD, et al. Elevated intra-abdominal pressure and renal function. Ann Surg 1982;196:594–7.
21. Sugrue M, Jones F, Deane SA, et al. Intra-abdominal hypertension is an independent cause of postoperative renal impairment. Arch Surg 1999;134:1082–5.
22. Bradley SE, Bradley GP. The effect of increased intra-abdominal pressure on renal function in man. J Clin Invest 1947;26:1010–22.
23. Bloomfield GL, Blocher CR, Fakhry IF, et al. Elevated intra-abdominal pressure increases plasma renin activity and aldosterone levels. J Trauma 1997;42: 997–1004 [discussion: 1005].
24. Diebel LN, Dulchavsky SA, Wilson RF. Effect of increased intra-abdominal pressure on mesenteric arterial and intestinal mucosal blood flow. J Trauma 1992; 33:45–8 [discussion: 48–9].
25. Burchard KW, Ciombor DM, McLeod MK, et al. Positive end expiratory pressure with increased intra-abdominal pressure. Surg Gynecol Obstet 1985;161:313–8.
26. Bongard F, Pianim N, Dubecz S, et al. Adverse consequences of increased intra-abdominal pressure on bowel tissue oxygen. J Trauma 1995;39:519–24 [discussion: 524–5].
27. Diebel LN, Dulchavsky SA, Brown WJ. Splanchnic ischemia and bacterial translocation in the abdominal compartment syndrome. J Trauma 1997;43:852–5.
28. Al-Dorzi HM, Tamim HM, Rishu AH, et al. Intra-abdominal pressure and abdominal perfusion pressure in cirrhotic patients with septic shock. Ann Intensive Care 2012;2(Suppl 1):S4.
29. De Waele JJ, Hoste EA, Malbrain ML. Decompressive laparotomy for abdominal compartment syndrome–a critical analysis. Crit Care 2006;10:R51.
30. Lee SL, Anderson JT, Kraut EJ, et al. A simplified approach to the diagnosis of elevated intra-abdominal pressure. J Trauma 2002;52:1169–72.
31. Sugrue M, Buist MD, Lee A, et al. Intra-abdominal pressure measurement using a modified nasogastric tube: description and validation of a new technique. Intensive Care Med 1994;20:588–90.
32. Malbrain ML. Different techniques to measure intra-abdominal pressure (IAP): time for a critical re-appraisal. Intensive Care Med 2004;30:357–71.
33. Cheatham ML, White MW, Sagraves SG, et al. Abdominal perfusion pressure: a superior parameter in the assessment of intra-abdominal hypertension. J Trauma 2000;49:621–6 [discussion: 626–7].
34. De Laet I, Hoste E, Verholen E, et al. The effect of neuromuscular blockers in patients with intra-abdominal hypertension. Intensive Care Med 2007;33:1811–4.
35. Corcos AC, Sherman HF. Percutaneous treatment of secondary abdominal compartment syndrome. J Trauma 2001;51:1062–4.
36. Savino JA, Cerabona T, Agarwal N, et al. Manipulation of ascitic fluid pressure in cirrhotics to optimize hemodynamic and renal function. Ann Surg 1988;208:504–11.

37. Sola-Vera J, Minana J, Ricart E, et al. Randomized trial comparing albumin and saline in the prevention of paracentesis-induced circulatory dysfunction in cirrhotic patients with ascites. Hepatology 2003;37:1147–53.
38. Vila MC, Sola R, Molina L, et al. Hemodynamic changes in patients developing effective hypovolemiá after total paracentesis. J Hepatol 1998;28:639–45.

# Nonvariceal Upper Gastrointestinal Bleeding

Syed Irfan-Ur Rahman, MD[a], Kia Saeian, MD, MSc Epi[b,*]

**KEYWORDS**

- Nonvariceal upper gastrointestinal bleed • Blatchford score • Rockall score
- Proton pump inhibitor • Nonsteroidal antiinflammatory drugs • Peptic ulcer disease
- Endoscopy

**KEY POINTS**

- Nonvariceal upper gastrointestinal bleeds are a medical emergency.
- The Blatchford and Rockall scores are useful risk stratification models.
- Nonvariceal upper gastrointestinal bleeding requires prompt assessment of respiratory status and hemodynamics, with prompt fluid resuscitation and blood product transfusions if necessary, and timely endoscopy.
- Proton pump inhibitors are the mainstay of pharmacologic treatment in nonvariceal upper gastrointestinal bleeding.
- Management is predicated on endoscopic findings and subsequent diagnosis with endoscopic therapy.

## INTRODUCTION

Nonvariceal upper gastrointestinal bleeding (NVUGB) often requires aggressive care and monitoring in the critical care setting. Several risk factors and models have been identified to guide clinical practice. Clinical features, including history and physical examination, provide important cues to ascertain a diagnosis and institute treatment. Physicians should be adept at developing a focused differential diagnosis to coordinate symptoms with disease processes. The primary goal is hemodynamic stability with fluid resuscitation and blood or blood product transfusions if warranted. Once this primary goal is achieved, pharmacologic therapy and endoscopic evaluation should follow. Urgent risk stratification, prompt hemodynamic stabilization, and endoscopic evaluation and identification of the bleeding source guide further management.

Disclosure: The authors have nothing to disclose.

[a] Department of Medicine, Medical College of Wisconsin, 9200 West Wisconsin Avenue, Milwaukee, WI 53226, USA; [b] Division of Gastroenterology and Hepatology, Department of Medicine, Medical College of Wisconsin, 9200 West Wisconsin Avenue, Milwaukee, WI 53226, USA
* Corresponding author.
*E-mail address:* ksaeian@mcw.edu

Crit Care Clin 32 (2016) 223–239
http://dx.doi.org/10.1016/j.ccc.2015.12.002
criticalcare.theclinics.com
0749-0704/16/$ – see front matter 

## EPIDEMIOLOGY

Gastrointestinal bleeding can be divided into upper and lower gastrointestinal bleeds with upper gastrointestinal bleeding (UGIB) defined as bleeding from a source proximal to the ligament of Treitz.[1] The annual rate of hospitalization and mortality for UGIB from 1992 to 1999 in the United States ranged from 172 per 100,000 to 149 per 100,000, and 10.9 per 100,000 to 7.8 per 100,000, respectively.[2] In general, the incidence of UGIB has steadily declined; however, the mortality remains stable. For example, from 1993 to 2000 the incidence of UGIBs declined by 23%. This decline is largely attributed to the treatment of *Helicobacter pylori* infection and use of acid-suppressive therapy for peptic ulcer disease (PUD).[3,4] Recent trends show that increased anticoagulation usage has not necessarily affected the incidence of NVUGB; however, the severity of bleeding episodes has worsened.[5] The incidence of NVUGB by diagnosis is documented in **Table 1**.[6]

## PATIENT EVALUATION OVERVIEW

### *Approach to the Upper Gastrointestinal Bleed*

A thorough history is vital in determining the cause, acuity, and volume loss following a UGIB. History should begin with an inquiry into the site, time frame, frequency, and intensity of UGIB. It is relevant to distinguish between UGIBs described by hematemesis, coffee-ground emesis, and melena caused by delayed transit of blood compared with lower gastrointestinal bleeding. Relevant past medical history, such as liver disease, PUD, inflammatory bowel disease, Peutz-Jeghers syndrome, and malignancy, have a propensity for gastrointestinal bleeds. Pertinent surgical history includes gastrectomy and abdominal aortic aneurysm repair. Medications should be reviewed for the use of nonsteroidal antiinflammatory drugs (NSAIDs), aspirin, anticoagulants, and antiplatelet agents. In addition, a family history of coagulation disorders may suggest underlying coagulation deficiencies, or a history of recurrent bleeding may suggest hereditary hemorrhagic telangiectasia. A retrospective study identified several clinical variables predictive of UGIB. **Table 2** details pertinent variables that increased the likelihood of UGIB. A Blatchford score of 0 (described later) decreases the likelihood that a UGIB requires intervention.[7]

Anemia and hypovolemia often occur concomitantly. Physicians should recognize signs of hypovolemia, including tachycardia, orthostatic hypotension, and an increased blood urea nitrogen/creatinine ratio. On examination, the color tint of the

**Table 1**
**Incidence of nonvariceal UGIB**

| Diagnosis | Incidence (%) |
|---|---|
| Peptic ulcer | 20–50 |
| Mallory-Weiss tear | 15–20 |
| Erosive gastritis/duodenitis | 10–15 |
| Esophagitis/esophageal ulcer | 5–10 |
| Malignancy | 1–2 |
| Angiodysplasia/vascular malformations | 5 |
| Other | 5 |

*From* Ferguson CB, Mitchell RM. Non-variceal upper gastrointestinal bleeding. Ulster Med J 2006;75(1):32–9.

**Table 4**
**Forrest classification**

| Class of Endoscopic Stigmata | Rebleeding Rate Without Therapy (%) |
|---|---|
| Type Ia: active arterial bleeding/spurting | 100 |
| Type Ib: oozing hemorrhage (without visible vessel) | 10–27 |
| Type IIa: nonbleeding visible vessel | Up to 50 |
| Type IIb: nonbleeding adherent clot | 8–35 |
| Type IIc: black/pigmented flat spot | <8 |
| Type III: clean ulcer base | <3 |

**Goals of resuscitation** Fluid resuscitation remains the cornerstone of hemodynamic management. It is imperative to rapidly restore circulating volume and correct tissue oxygen deficits. Resuscitation and attempts to control the source of ongoing gastrointestinal blood loss should ideally occur simultaneously because resuscitation is unlikely to be successful, especially with incessant hemorrhage. Crystalloid solutions are generally preferred as the immediate modality of administration of resuscitation volume. However over-resuscitation with intravenous fluids may contribute to the development of complications such as coagulopathy, tissue edema, and pulmonary edema.[17,18] Thus, although fluid resuscitation remains the first-line therapy for restoration of intravascular volume, resuscitation needs to be optimized with consideration given to ongoing hemorrhage, strategies for definitive therapy, coagulopathy, and close hemodynamic monitoring. There is intense debate over target blood pressure values in acutely bleeding patients without trauma. Although guidelines for bleeding patients with trauma suggest maintaining a systolic blood pressure between 80 and 90 mm Hg, there remains a paucity of literature in the nontrauma population.[19,20] From a physiologic standpoint for ongoing hemorrhage, the authors suggest accepting lower blood pressures if tissue perfusion is maintained. Moreover, in these cases, control of hemorrhage as quickly as possible remains a priority.

**Transfusion strategies** Resuscitation with blood is lifesaving in the setting of exsanguination and is sometimes required to restore red cell oxygen carrying capacity. Strategies for resuscitation of massively hemorrhaging patients and the use of massive

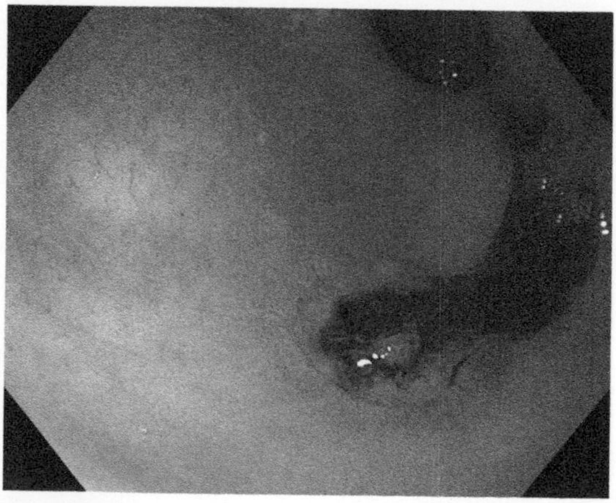

**Fig. 1.** Bleeding visible vessel.

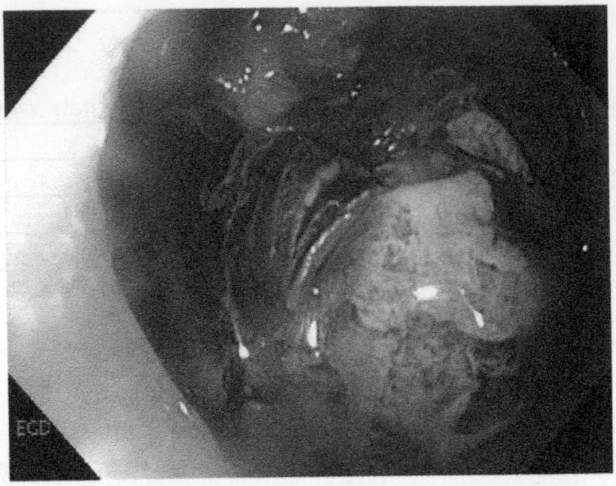


**Fig. 2.** Ulcer with clot.

transfusion protocols have been the focus of the trauma literature for the past decade.[21] Extrapolated from a concept first introduced in military practice, fixed ratio packed red cell (PRBC) to other blood component resuscitation has now been widely adopted in civilian trauma as well.[22,23] This fixed ratio resuscitation strategy incorporates hemostatic resuscitation with the use of PRBC, fresh frozen plasma, and platelet in a 1:1:1 ratio. This strategy seems to lessen acute traumatic coagulopathy, the presence of which is associated with significant increases in mortality and morbidity. Massive transfusion has traditionally been defined as the requirement of 10 or more units of PRBC in a period of 24 hours. However, by identifying patients who needed more than 3 units of PRBC per hour, Savage and colleagues[24] were able to predict mortality more accurately than the traditional definition of massive transfusion. It is important to recognize that this strategy was designed for the resuscitation of patients with trauma and the outcomes or applicability of this to patients without trauma is currently unknown. However, most hospitals have massive transfusion protocols and the fixed ratio approach is used for bleeding patients without trauma as well, despite the lack of evidence, because it seems physiologically sound. The authors suggest that consideration be given to replacement of plasma and platelets when more than 3 to 4 units of PRBC are rapidly required to stabilize a patient with UGIB.

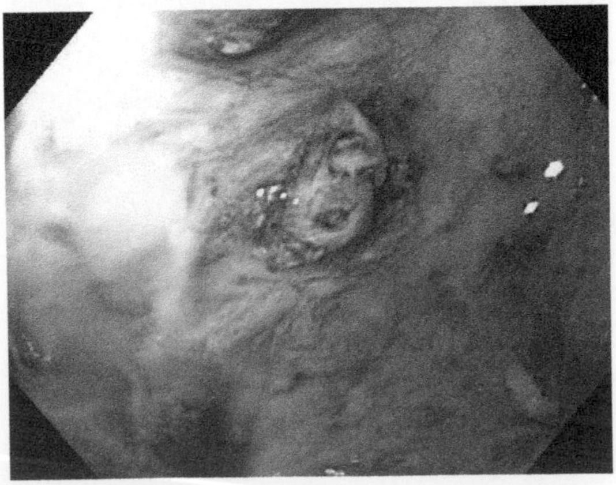

**Fig. 3.** Ulcer after clot removed.

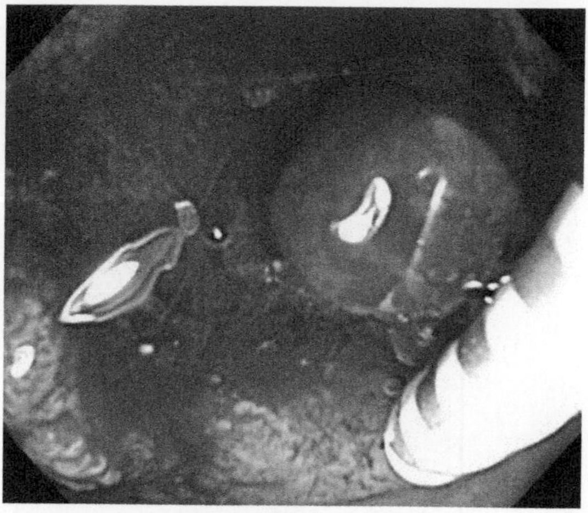

**Fig. 4.** Bleeding ulcer treated with gold probe.

For patients without brisk bleeding, the optimal hemoglobin target is controversial. A landmark study that randomized patients with UGIB to a restrictive transfusion strategy (trigger for transfusion: hemoglobin level <7 g/dL) versus a liberal strategy (trigger for transfusion: hemoglobin level <9 g/dL) showed that the restrictive strategy significantly improved outcomes. Patients in the restrictive strategy group were less likely to die at 6 weeks and had lesser rebleeding rates. Even when the analysis was restricted to patients with only PUD, although not statistically significant, the signal still favored the restrictive strategy group. Note that this study excluded patients with exsanguination and acute coronary syndromes. Nevertheless, this study suggests that, in the appropriate patient population and in the absence of hemodynamic instability or massive bleeding, a restrictive transfusion strategy is safe.[25]

**Correction of coagulopathy** UGIB often occurs in the setting of coagulopathy, which typically requires immediate correction with fresh frozen plasma, platelets, cryoprecipitate, or a combination thereof. Vitamin K may be given to reverse

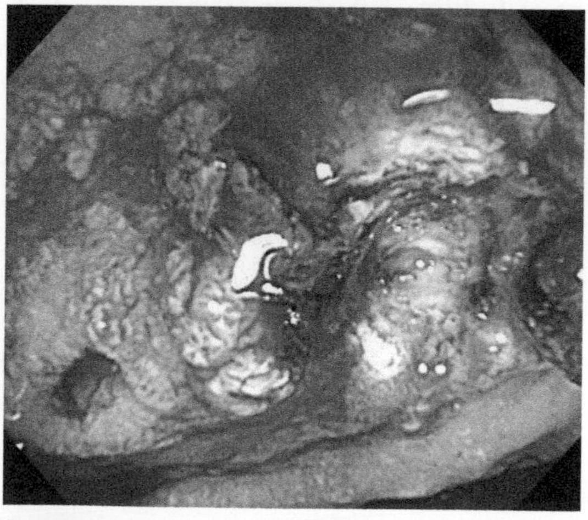

**Fig. 5.** Ulcer after therapy.

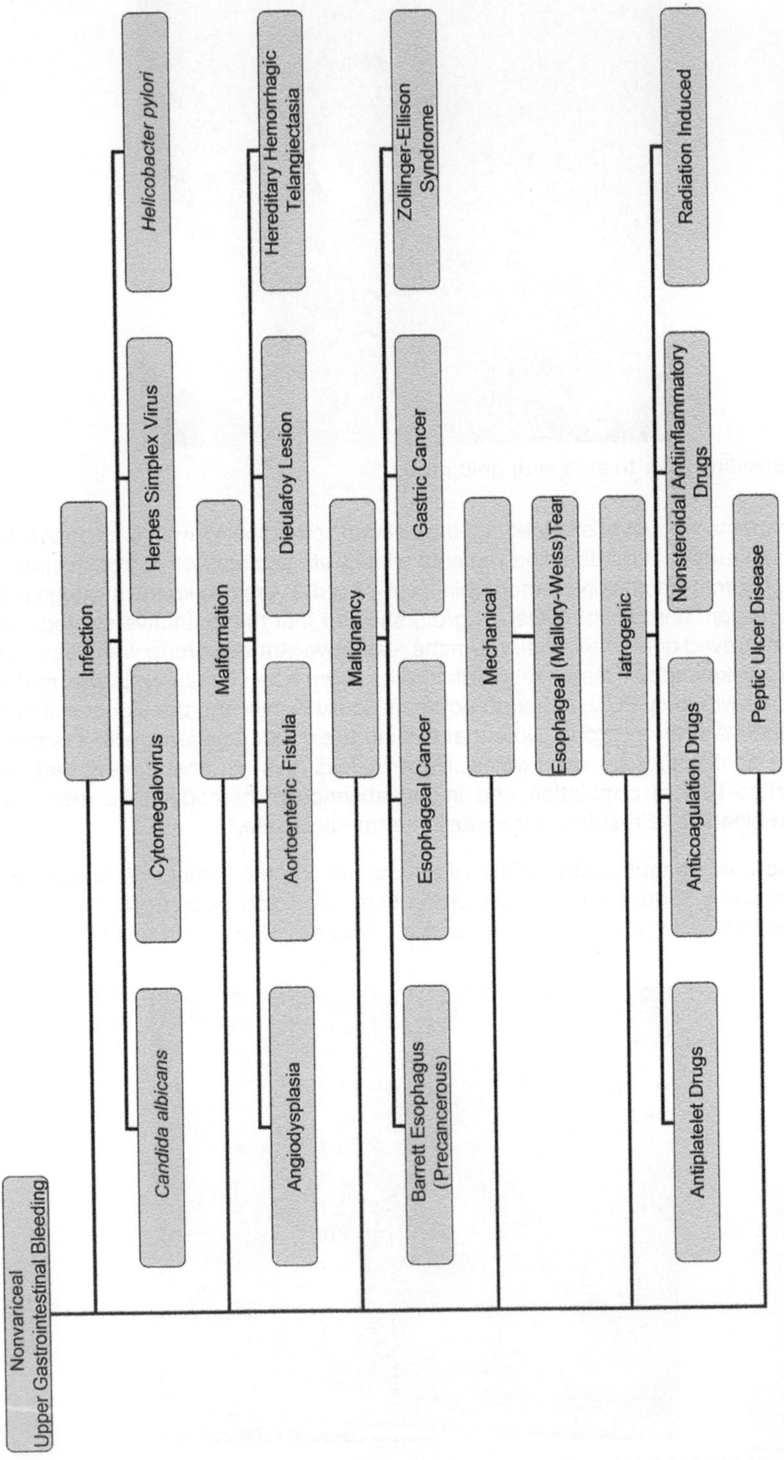


**Fig. 6.** Differential diagnosis of nonvariceal upper gastrointestinal bleeds.

**Table 5**
**Stepwise evaluation of NVUGB**

| Priority | Action |
|---|---|
| 1 | Assess patient and ensure adequate airway, check respiration, and obtain vital signs (including orthostatics) |
| 2 | Perform focused physical examination including digital rectal examination unless stool evident |
| 3 | Infuse rapid bolus of fluids based on hemodynamic status |
| 4 | Establish 2 large bore IV access |
| 5 | Order stat laboratory tests (complete blood count, liver enzymes, coagulation studies, creatinine, and blood urea nitrogen) |
| 6 | Transfusion parameters<br>a. Hemoglobin level <7 g/dL (70 g/L) in low-risk patients[15,16]<br>b. Platelet counts for thrombocytopenia (platelet count <50,000/mL)<br>c. Fresh frozen plasma for coagulopathy; however, should not delay endoscopy[16] |
| 7 | Gastroenterology consultation for endoscopic evaluation |
| 8 | Proton pump inhibitor therapy and consider prokinetics |

*Abbreviation:* IV, intravenous.

warfarin-associated coagulopathy but this usually takes a few hours. If used, vitamin K should be given intravenously to ensure rapidity of onset of action. Although common practice is to use the prothrombin time (PT) or partial thromboplastin time (PTT) as a guide to correction of the hemostatic defect, there is a current trend toward using viscoelastic testing (thromboelastography or rotation thromboelastometry) to guide resuscitation because PT and PTT may not accurately reflect the underlying hemostatic defect and do not provide information about platelet function, clot strength, and fibrinolysis, all of which are disadvantages that are overcome by viscoelastic testing.[26] Use of viscoelastic testing has the potential to provide dynamic assessment of coagulation, optimize blood product use, and minimize overtransfusion.

If there is anticipation of the need for large volumes of blood products to reverse coagulopathy and there is a concern for timeliness of reversal of unwanted side effects such as volume overload, consideration may be given to transfusion of newer products, such prothrombin complex concentrates. These newer products may also be necessary to reverse coagulopathy associated with newer anticoagulant agents other than warfarin.

***Pharmacologic treatment options***

The standard of care for NVUGB is proton pump inhibitor (PPI) therapy. A Cochran Systematic Review showed that preendoscopic PPI-treated patients maintained a reduced need for endoscopic surveillance as well as fewer high-risk stigmata compared with a control group receiving placebo or a histamine 2 receptor antagonist. Of note, this study showed that PPI therapy before endoscopy failed to show statistical significance in major end points, specifically mortality, rebleeding, and need for operative intervention.[27] It is recommended to offer an intravenous bolus followed by twice-daily PPI (initially intravenous and subsequently oral when feasible), with continuous-infusion PPI therapy reserved for those having undergone endoscopic therapy to decrease rebleeding and mortality in patients with high-risk stigmata following endoscopic therapy. Both intravenous and oral PPI therapy have also been shown to decrease the length of hospital stay, rebleeding rate, and need for blood transfusion in patients with high-risk ulcers treated with endoscopic therapy.

The use of histamine 2 receptor antagonists, somatostatin, and octreotide is not routinely recommended for NVUGBs.[16]

Pharmacologic treatment may also be used as an adjunct to endoscopy. Prokinetic agents (eg, erythromycin 3 mg/kg intravenously over 20–30 minutes, 30–60 minutes before endoscopy) seem to enhance the rate of adequate endoscopic visualization and decrease the need for second-look endoscopy. However, in the absence of significantly improved definitive end points (eg, mortality, transfusion requirement), routine use of prokinetic medications is not recommended; the authors typically use erythromycin if significant gastric residue is suspected.[28,29]

**Chronic management** Special attention is required in patients who require antiplatelet therapy. In patients with a documented bleeding ulcer who require NSAIDs, a combination of a PPI and cyclooxygenase-2 inhibitor is warranted. As a corollary in patients with documented bleeding ulcer who require aspirin for cardiovascular prophylaxis, a risk and benefit analysis should be discussed with the patient.[16] Note that a randomized control trial showed that clopidogrel had a higher risk of rebleeding compared with aspirin plus PPI.[30] A multidisciplinary approach to those requiring antiplatelet agents in the setting of NVUGB is helpful in addressing the most prudent therapy.

***Nonpharmacologic treatment options***

Appropriate management of NVUGB requires hospitals to maintain institutional protocols and a multidisciplinary team with access to a trained endoscopist. Early endoscopy, defined as being performed within 24 hours of presentation, should be undertaken after or, if necessary, in conjunction with hemodynamic stabilization, although definitive data on improved hard outcomes such as mortality are lacking.[31] Early endoscopy (within 24 hours) does facilitate early discharge of low-risk patients and may improve outcomes in high-risk patients.[32] Although one meta-analysis found no difference in outcomes comparing very early endoscopy (<12 hours) with early endoscopy (<24 hours), another study found less need for blood transfusions and decreased length of hospital stay in patients with blood in gastric tube aspirate if endoscopy was performed in less than 12 hours compared with more than 12 hours.[33] These divergent results are likely caused by the heterogeneity of patient populations included in the studies and, because of their time frame (many completed >20 years ago), should be cautiously applied to current management strategies. Adamopoulos and colleagues[34] identified fresh blood in the nasogastric tube aspirate, hemodynamic instability, hemoglobin level less than 8 g/dL, and a leukocyte count of more than 12,000/mL as independent predictors of the need for endoscopy within 12 hours of presentation. Although not conclusive, this suggests that timing of endoscopy should be individualized and the presence of high-risk characteristics should add impetus to earlier endoscopy. In addition to allowing definitive diagnosis and appropriate stratification, endoscopy allows the use of multiple techniques, including injection therapy (eg, epinephrine), often in concert with hemoclips, cautery via thermal or electrical conduction (most often via bipolar coagulation probe), sclerosant agents, argon plasma coagulation, and band ligation in NVUGB (**Table 6**). Endoscopic treatments are often disease specific, with the most definitive data available for PUD. A study to evaluate hemostatic efficacy compared bipolar hemostatic forceps and hemoclip use by dividing patients into group I and II to treat NVUGBs, respectively. The time required to achieve hemostasis was 6.8 ± 13.4 minutes for group I and 15.4 ± 17.0 minutes for group II. In addition, 100% of patients in group I compared with 78.2% patients in group II reached hemostasis, suggesting that bipolar hemostatic forceps are more efficacious than hemoclip use.[35]

**Table 6**
**Endoscopic techniques**

| Endoscopy Technique | Mechanism of Action |
|---|---|
| Injection (epinephrine) | Volume effect producing local tamponade |
| Sclerosant | Direct tissue injury and thrombosis |
| Cautery | Mechanical pressure producing local tamponade combined with heat or electrical current to coagulate blood vessels; known as coaptation |
| Thrombin/fibrin/ cyanoacrylate glue | Primary tissue seal at bleeding site |
| Argon plasma coagulation | Ionized gas to conduct electricity, resulting in coagulation |
| Clip and/or band ligation | Physical effect producing tamponade |

Overall, initial hemostasis is successful in expert hands in most cases. During endoscopy, on discovery of a clot, vigorous irrigation is necessary to expose an underlying ulcer bed. However, adherent clots require endoscopic therapy if high risk (epinephrine preinjection and shaving via cold guillotining snare technique of the clot to expose the underlying vessel) and, if low risk and/or endoscopic therapy is not feasible, then PPI therapy based on a randomized control trial.[36] Routine secondary endoscopies are not recommended. If there is evidence of continued or recurrent bleeding, a second-look endoscopy for continued evidence of bleeding is warranted and, if attempts at treatment fail, then along with surgical consultation percutaneous embolization should be considered, especially in nonsurgical candidates.[37,38] Following endoscopic hemostasis, which is successful at initial hemostasis in most cases, patient disposition primarily depends on risk of rebleeding as dictated by the endoscopic findings (see **Table 4**) along with the patient's clinical status. In simple terms, select patients with acute UGIB with low risk of rebleed may be discharged promptly, whereas those with high-risk endoscopic stigmata require 72 hours of hospitalization.[16] A simplified approach to endoscopic evaluation is shown in **Fig. 7**.

***Disease-specific treatment options***

**Infection** Infections of the esophagus can be a product of cytomegalovirus, herpes simplex virus, and *Candida albicans*. Affected patients are typically immunocompromised and present with odynophagia and dysphagia; NVUGB reflects a severe case. Diagnosis is established by endoscopy findings and histologic examination. Findings including treatment options are summarized in **Table 7**.

*H pylori* infection is associated with gastric ulcers, duodenal ulcers, gastric cancer, and mucosa-associated lymphoid tissue lymphoma. Presence of gastric erythema consistent with gastritis may be suggestive. Diagnostic tests include endoscopic biopsy or urease testing, urease breath tests, stool antigen assay, and serologies. Of note, serology cannot distinguish between active and prior infections. All patients with PUD should be tested for *H pylori* infection with repeat interval testing if the patient is at high risk for false-negatives (eg, recent antibiotic and/or PPI use at time of biopsy). The reasonable first-line regimen for *H pylori* is triple therapy with PPI, amoxicillin, and clarithromycin. In areas of high antibiotic resistance, quadruple therapy with PPI, bismuth subsalicylate, metronidazole, and tetracycline is recommended. Treatment failures require alternative triple or quadruple regimens. Eradication should be confirmed by urea breath test or stool antigen assay based on facility preference in all cases of significant UGIB.

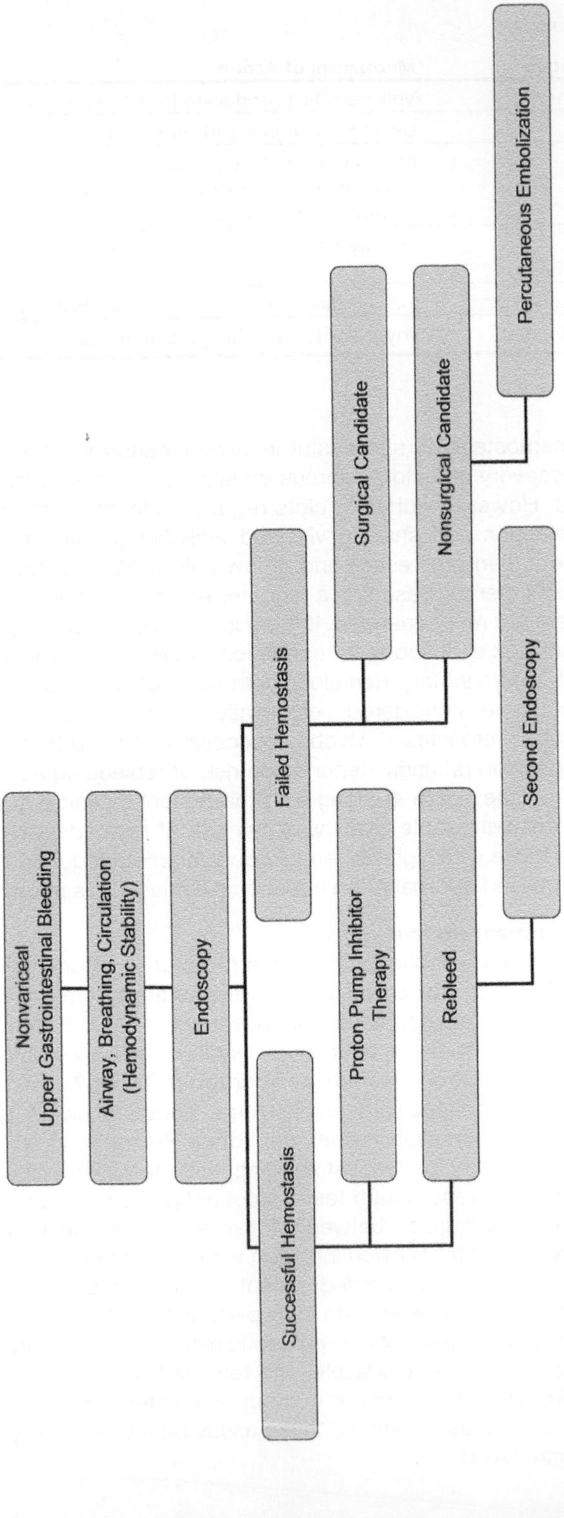


**Fig. 7.** Stepwise endoscopic evaluation.

**Table 7**
**Infectious esophagitis**

| Diagnosis | Endoscopy | Histology | Treatment |
|---|---|---|---|
| *C albicans* | Pseudomembranous or white covered plaques | Yeast and/or pseudohyphae | 1. Fluconazole<br>2. Other azoles<br>3. Echinocandins or amphotericin B |
| Cytomegalovirus | Large ulcers/erosions | Inclusions bodies or Owl's eyes | Patient specific; eg, ganciclovir |
| Herpes simplex virus | Multiple well-defined shallow ulcers/erosions | Eosinophilic inclusions (Cowdry A), multinucleated giant cells, and ground-glass nuclei | 1. Acyclovir<br>2. Famciclovir or valacyclovir |

**Malformation** Arteriovenous malformations are vascular anomalies in direct connection between arteries and veins without a capillary bed. They can be seen in angiodysplasia or in concert with syndromes such as hereditary hemorrhagic telangiectasia. Dieulafoy lesion is a vascular anomaly that represents caliber persistent arteries that may rupture causing massive bleed, often in the proximal stomach although they may occur in other parts of the GI tract. These lesions may be difficult to identify, requiring a knowledgeable endoscopist and some good fortune and timing. Gastric antral vascular ectasia (GAVE), also known as watermelon stomach, is a collection of dilated vessels treated with endothermal ablation or antrectomy. This entity results in more chronic blood loss, or at least low-volume blood loss. In addition, a history of an aortic aneurysm repair should highlight the possibility of an aortoenteric fistula often 3 to 5 years following reconstructive surgery (native fistulas in the absence of a repair are exceedingly rare). In general, endoscopic therapy for these entities are individualized based on the specific lesion, but cautery via bipolar coagulation and argon plasma coagulation is most frequently used. Alternative treatments include operative intervention or angiography in nonsurgical candidates who fail endoscopic therapy.

**Malignancy** NVUGB is a common clinical manifestation in both esophageal and gastric cancers. For esophageal cancer, risks factors for adenocarcinoma (Barrett esophagus) and squamous cell carcinoma (tobacco smoking and alcohol usage) may provide clues in the setting of NVUGB. A wider range of risk factors are associated with gastric adenocarcinoma (eg, *H pylori* infection, atrophic gastritis, prior gastric surgery, a diet high in nitroso compounds among other risk factors). Endoscopy may be diagnostic via tissue biopsy and may offer therapeutic options, particularly in patients with obstructive symptoms (eg, luminal stents in esophageal cancer) in addition to temporizing bleeding, although endoscopic bleeding control in such settings is suboptimal.

**Mechanical** Mallory-Weiss tear is a potential life-threatening condition caused by a sudden increase in intra-abdominal pressure resulting in acute NVUGBs. Causes include vomiting, retching, severe coughing, and trauma often in the setting of chronic alcohol use. Endoscopy is the test of choice both for diagnosis and therapeutic hemostasis. All techniques, including local injection, hemoclip, multipolar electrocoagulation, and endoscopic band ligation, are equally effective. These varied approaches are recommended based on presence or absence of hemorrhage and endoscopist expertise.[39]

**Iatrogenic** There are several iatrogenic causes of NVUGB, including NSAID/antiplatelet therapy (discussed earlier, and by far the most common) and direct trauma from instrumentation such as nasogastric tubes.

**Peptic ulcer disease** PUD is often asymptomatic, but can manifest as dyspepsia, abdominal pain, early satiety, nausea, and vomiting. Causative agents of PUD include NSAIDs/antiplatelet agents, *H pylori* infection, corticosteroid use in conjunction with antiplatelet therapy, hypersecretory syndromes, viral diseases, vascular insufficiency, and chemoradiation and/or radiation therapy. Complicated PUD is defined by overt bleeding as well as obstruction, perforation, and potentially fistula formation. A diagnostic evaluation is largely based on endoscopy to delineate the size; characteristics, including risk stigmata; and histopathology via biopsy of the ulcer (particularly gastric ulcers, which potentially harbor malignancy). Bleeding ulcers are treated with endoscopy; specifically epinephrine injections, hemoclip use, thermal coagulation, or interventional angiography, or operatively with either resection with or without vagotomy or an omental (Graham) patch. The long-term management of PUD consists of testing and treating for *H pylori* infection as well as PPI therapy. There is no difference between oral and intravenous PPI in terms of recurrent bleeding, mean volume of blood transfused, need for surgery, or all-cause mortality.[40] However, intravenous PPIs achieve an intragastric pH less than 6 faster than oral agents.[41] In addition, recent studies have proposed that intermittent PPI therapy is not inferior to continuous PPI therapy as earlier literature may have suggested.[42]

***Special consideration***

Left ventricular assist devices (LVADs) are advanced heart failure tools that assist in patients with severe congestive heart failure. NVUGB is a common complication among patients with LVADs. Theories to explain this association include Hedye syndrome, von Willebrand factor breakdown via mechanical disruption, proximity of the celiac trunk to the LVAD, and LVAD pump speeds in patients with weakened vasculature. Risk factors for NVUGBs in patients with LVADs include right ventricular dysfunction, renal dysfunction, and post-LVAD ejection fraction greater than 30%. Endoscopy is the treatment of choice in patients with LVADs presenting with NVUGB to identify a source of bleed and provide hemostasis, although this can be difficult, especially in the setting of the continued need for anticoagulation and antiplatelet therapy. Frequently, multiple additional tests, including colonoscopy, video capsule endoscopy, antegrade enteroscopy, angiography, and nuclear medicine tagged red blood cell scans, may also be required.[43]

## FUTURE DIRECTION

Emerging endoscopic techniques have been developed for NVUGB. Novel endoscopic methods to achieve hemostasis include over-the-counter scope clips, hemostatic sprays, cryotherapy, radiofrequency ablation, endoscopic suturing, and endoscopic ultrasonography–guided angiotherapy. Their clinical application, although not currently widespread, is promising and is enumerated along with their limitations in **Table 8**.[44]

These methods may be used as primary or rescue therapy. Further studies are needed to evaluate the indication, safety, and efficacy of these novel endoscopic techniques.

**Table 8**
**Emerging endoscopic techniques**

| Endoscopic Technique | Clinical Application | Limitation |
|---|---|---|
| Over-the-counter scope clips | NVUGBs refractory to standard therapies | Cost, device manipulation |
| Hemostatic sprays | Oozing lesions | Washes away in brisk bleeds |
| Cryotherapy | GAVE | Requires multiple treatments |
| Radiofrequency ablation | GAVE | Technical dexterity with catheter manipulation |
| Endoscopic suturing | Chronic blood loss resulting from anastomotic ulcers | Technical complexity in active bleeding |
| Endoscopic ultrasonography–guided angiotherapy | Varices | Endosonographer training, limited availability of sonography |

## REFERENCES


1. Wilcox CM, Alexander LN, Cotsonis G. A prospective characterization of upper gastrointestinal hemorrhage presenting with hematochezia. Am J Gastroenterol 1997;92:231–5.
2. Lewis JD, Bilker WB, Brensinger C, et al. Hospitalization and mortality rates from peptic ulcer disease and GI bleeding in the 1990s: relationship to sales of nonsteroidal anti-inflammatory drugs and acid suppression medications. Am J Gastroenterol 2002;97(10):2540–9.
3. Targownik LE, Nabalamba A. Trends in management and outcomes of acute nonvariceal upper gastrointestinal bleeding: 1993-2003. Clin Gastroenterol Hepatol 2006;4(12):1459–66.
4. Van Leerdam ME, Vreeburg EM, Rauws EA, et al. Acute upper GI bleeding: did anything change? Time trend analysis of incidence and outcome of acute upper GI bleeding between 1993/1994 and 2000. Am J Gastroenterol 2003;98(7):1494–9.
5. Ahsberg K, Höglund P, Kim WH, et al. Impact of aspirin, NSAIDs, warfarin, corticosteroids and SSRIs on the site and outcome of non-variceal upper and lower gastrointestinal bleeding. Scand J Gastroenterol 2010;45(12):1404–15.
6. Ferguson CB, Mitchell RM. Non-variceal upper gastrointestinal bleeding. Ulster Med J 2006;75(1):32–9.
7. Srygley FD, Gerardo CJ, Tran T, et al. Does this patient have a severe upper gastrointestinal bleed? JAMA 2012;307(10):1072–9.
8. Strobach RS, Anderson SK, Doll DC, et al. The value of the physical examination in the diagnosis of anemia. Correlation of the physical findings and the hemoglobin concentration. Arch Intern Med 1988;148(4):831–2.
9. Witting MD, Magder L, Heins AE, et al. Usefulness and validity of diagnostic nasogastric aspiration in patients without hematemesis. Ann Emerg Med 2004;43(4):525–32.
10. Blatchford O, Murray WR, Blatchford M. A risk score to predict need for treatment for upper-gastrointestinal haemorrhage. Lancet 2000;356:1318–21.
11. Rockall TA, Logan RF, Devlin HB, et al. Risk assessment after acute upper gastrointestinal haemorrhage. Gut 1996;38:316–21.
12. Wang CH, Chen YW, Young YR, et al. A prospective comparison of 3 scoring systems in upper gastrointestinal bleeding. Am J Emerg Med 2013;31(5):775–8.

13. Chen IC, Hung MS, Chiu TF, et al. Risk scoring systems to predict need for clinical intervention for patients with nonvariceal upper gastrointestinal tract bleeding. Am J Emerg Med 2007;25(7):774–9.
14. Forrest JA, Finlayson ND, Shearman DJ. Endoscopy in gastrointestinal bleeding. Lancet 1974;2:394–7.
15. Hébert PC, Wells G, Blajchman MA, et al. A multicenter, randomized, controlled clinical trial of transfusion requirements in critical care. Transfusion Requirements in Critical Care Investigators, Canadian Critical Care Trials Group. N Engl J Med 1999;340:409–17.
16. Barkun AN, Bardou M, Kuipers EJ, et al. International consensus recommendations on the management of patients with nonvariceal upper gastro-intestinal bleeding. Ann Intern Med 2010;152:101–13.
17. Boyd JH, Forbes J, Nakada TA, et al. Fluid resuscitation in septic shock: a positive fluid balance and elevated central venous pressure are associated with increased mortality. Crit Care Med 2011;39(2):259–65.
18. Bellomo R, Cass A, Cole L, et al. An observational study fluid balance and patient outcomes in the Randomized Evaluation of Normal vs. Augmented Level of Replacement Therapy trial. Crit Care Med 2012;40(6):1753–60.
19. Dutton RP, Mackenzie CF, Scalea TM. Hypotensive resuscitation during active hemorrhage: impact on in-hospital mortality. J Trauma 2002;52(6):1141–6.
20. Spahn DR, Bouillon B, Cerny V, et al. Management of bleeding and coagulopathy following major trauma: an updated European guideline. Crit Care 2013;17(2):R76.
21. Neal MD, Marsh A, Marino R, et al. Massive transfusion: an evidence-based review of recent developments. Arch Surg 2012;147(6):563–71.
22. Borgman MA, Spinella PC, Perkins JG, et al. The ratio of blood products transfused affects mortality in patients receiving massive transfusions at a combat support hospital. J Trauma 2007;63(4):805–13.
23. Holcomb JB, del Junco DJ, Fox EE, et al. The Prospective, Observational, Multicenter, Major Trauma Transfusion (PROMMTT) study: comparative effectiveness of a time-varying treatment with competing risks. JAMA Surg 2013;148(2):127–36.
24. Savage SA, Zarzaur BL, Croce MA, et al. Redefining massive transfusion when every second counts. J Trauma Acute Care Surg 2013;74(2):396–400.
25. Villanueva C, Colomo A, Bosch A, et al. Transfusion strategies for acute upper gastrointestinal bleeding. N Engl J Med 2013;368(1):11–21.
26. Dempfle CE, Borggrefe M. Point of care coagulation tests in critically ill patients [review]. Semin Thromb Hemost 2008;34(5):445–50.
27. Sreedharan A, Martin J, Leontiadis G, et al. Proton pump inhibitor treatment initiated prior to endoscopic diagnosis in upper gastrointestinal bleeding. Cochrane Database Syst Rev 2010;(7):CD005415.
28. Coffin B, Pocard M, Panis Y, et al. Erythromycin improves the quality of EGD in patients with acute upper GI bleeding: a randomized controlled study. Gastrointest Endosc 2002;56(2):174–9.
29. Frossard JL, Spahr L, Queneau PE, et al. Erythromycin intravenous bolus infusion in acute upper gastrointestinal bleeding: a randomized, controlled, double-blind trial. Gastroenterology 2002;123(1):17–23.
30. Lai KC, Chu KM, Hui WM, et al. Esomeprazole with aspirin versus clopidogrel for prevention of recurrent gastrointestinal ulcer complications. Clin Gastroenterol Hepatol 2006;4:860–5.
31. Spiegel BM, Vakil NB, Ofman JJ. Endoscopy for acute nonvariceal upper gastrointestinal tract hemorrhage: is sooner better? A systematic review. Arch Intern Med 2001;161:1393–404.

32. Jairath V, Kahan BC, Logan RF, et al. Outcomes following acute nonvariceal upper gastrointestinal bleeding in relation to time to endoscopy: results from a nationwide study. Endoscopy 2012;44(8):723–30.
33. Lin HJ, Wang K, Perng CL, et al. Early or delayed endoscopy for patients with peptic ulcer bleeding. A prospective randomized study. J Clin Gastroenterol 1996;22(4):267–71.
34. Adamopoulos AB, Baibas NM, Efstathiou SP, et al. Differentiation between patients with acute upper gastrointestinal bleeding who need early urgent upper gastrointestinal endoscopy and those who do not. A prospective study. Eur J Gastroenterol Hepatol 2003;15(4):381–7.
35. Kataoka M, Kawai T, Hayama Y, et al. Comparison of hemostasis using bipolar hemostatic forceps with hemostasis by endoscopic hemoclipping for nonvariceal upper gastrointestinal bleeding in a prospective non-randomized trial. Surg Endosc 2013;27(8):3035–8.
36. Sung JJ, Chan FK, Lau JY, et al. The effect of endoscopic therapy in patients receiving omeprazole for bleeding ulcers with nonbleeding visible vessels or adherent clots: a randomized comparison. Ann Intern Med 2003;139:237–43.
37. Kim S, Duddalwar V. Failed endoscopic therapy and the interventional radiologist: non-variceal upper gastrointestinal bleeding. Tech Gastrointest Endosc 2005;7:148–55.
38. Lau JY, Sung JJ, Lam YH, et al. Endoscopic retreatment compared with surgery in patients with recurrent bleeding after initial endoscopic control of bleeding ulcers. N Engl J Med 1999;340:751–6.
39. Yin A, Li Y, Jiang Y, et al. Mallory-Weiss syndrome: clinical and endoscopic characteristics. Eur J Intern Med 2012;23(4):e92–6.
40. Tsoi KK, Hirai HW, Sung JJ. Meta-analysis: comparison of oral vs. intravenous proton pump inhibitors in patients with peptic ulcer bleeding. Aliment Pharmacol Ther 2013;38(7):721–8.
41. Laine L, Shah A, Bemanian S. Intragastric pH with oral vs intravenous bolus plus infusion proton-pump inhibitor therapy in patients with bleeding ulcers. Gastroenterology 2008;134(7):1836.
42. Sachar H, Vaidya K, Laine L. Intermittent vs continuous proton pump inhibitor therapy for high-risk bleeding ulcers: a systematic review and meta-analysis. JAMA Intern Med 2014;174(11):1755.
43. Jabbar HR, Abbas A, Ahmed M, et al. The incidence, predictors and outcomes of gastrointestinal bleeding in patients with left ventricular assist device (LVAD). Dig Dis Sci 2015;60(12):3697–706.
44. Song LM, Levy MJ. Emerging endoscopic therapies for nonvariceal upper gastrointestinal bleeding. Gastroenterol Clin North Am 2014;43(4):721–37.

# Lower Gastrointestinal Hemorrhage

Emad Qayed, MD[a], Gaurav Dagar, MD[b], Rahul S. Nanchal, MD, MS[c,*]

**KEYWORDS**

• Lower gastrointestinal bleeding • Colonoscopy • Diverticulosis • Angiography

**KEY POINTS**

- Lower gastrointestinal bleeding (LGIB) is a frequent cause of hospitalization and admission to the intensive care unit (ICU) especially in the elderly patient.
- Approximately 11% of LGIB are secondary to brisk upper GI bleeding. Lower GI bleeds are usually less severe in nature than upper GI bleeds.
- Colonoscopy remains the most common modality for evaluating LGIB. Colonoscopy can be both diagnostic and therapeutic. The optimal timing of colonoscopy in a patient who presents with LGIB is controversial.
- Radionuclide studies, angiographic therapy and surgery are other localization and treatment options for LGIB where colonoscopy fails.
- Small bowel bleeds now considered a separate entity, usually present with hematochezia and are classified as obscure causes of LGIB. Angiodysplasias are the most common cause of small bowel or obscure bleeds. Wireless capsule endoscopy, push enteroscopy and deep enteroscopy are methods to evaluate the small bowel for bleeding.

Lower gastrointestinal bleeding (LGIB) is a frequent reason for hospitalization especially in the elderly. Patients with LGIB are frequently admitted to the intensive care unit and may require transfusion of packed red blood cells (PRBC) and other blood products especially in the setting of coagulopathy. Colonoscopy is often performed to localize the source of bleeding and sometimes provision of therapeutic measures, such as argon plasma coagulation. LGIB may present as an acute life-threatening event or as a chronic insidious condition manifesting as iron deficiency anemia and positivity for fecal occult blood. This article discusses the presentation, diagnosis, and management of LGIB with a focus on conditions that present with acute blood loss.

[a] Grady Memorial Hospital, Emory University School of Medicine, 49 Jesse Hill Junior Drive, Atlanta, GA 30303, USA; [b] Division of Pulmonary and Critical Care Medicine, Medical College of Wisconsin, Milwaukee, WI 53188, USA; [c] Critical Care Fellowship Program, Medical Intensive Care Unit, Division of Pulmonary and Critical Care Medicine, Suite E 5200, 9200 West Wisconsin Avenue, Milwaukee, WI 53226, USA
* Corresponding author.
*E-mail address:* Rnanchal@mcw.edu

Crit Care Clin 32 (2016) 241–254
http://dx.doi.org/10.1016/j.ccc.2015.12.004 criticalcare.theclinics.com

## DEFINITION

LGIB has traditionally been defined as that occurring beyond the ligament of Treitz.[1] Since the advent of capsule endoscopy and demonstration that small bowel bleeds are a separate clinical entity,[2] some authors define LGIB as blood loss from the colon and/or anorectum. LGIB may be acute or chronic, with acute typically denoting blood loss of recent duration (arbitrary value of <3 days) and chronic signaling blood loss over a longer duration, typically days to weeks. Acute LGIB is usually overt presenting with hematochezia or melena and may result in hemodynamic instability. Conversely, chronic LGIB is usually occult presenting as iron deficiency anemia and/or positive fecal occult blood testing.

## EPIDEMIOLOGY

Investigations pertaining to the epidemiology of LGIB are infrequent. Moreover, definitions and criteria of inclusion differ among studies leading to variable results. Nevertheless, LGIB represents approximately 20% to 25% of all cases with gastrointestinal (GI) bleeds.[3] This number is likely an underestimation because unlike upper GI bleeds (UGIB), many patients with milder forms of LGIB either do not present to the hospital or are not admitted. The annual incidence is estimated to be between 20 and 27 cases per 100,000 population.[4,5] The incidence increases with advancing age with a greater than 200-fold increase between the ages of 20 and 80.[4] LGIB also occurs more commonly in men than in women.[4] The increasing incidence with age is likely secondary to the increasing prevalence of diverticulosis and angiodysplasia with age, both common causes of LGIB. The associated mortality ranges from 2% to 4%[6] but may be significantly higher in elderly patients presenting with hemodynamic instability. One French prospective study identified 1333 patients with LGIB. In this study the mean age was 72 years and a predisposing medicine contributing to the LGIB was found in 75% of patients (antiplatelet agents, anti–vitamin K agents, nonsteroidal anti-inflammatory drugs [NSAIDs], and heparin).[7]

## CRITERIA FOR SEVERITY AND RISK STRATIFICATION

LGIB is usually slower and less severe than UGIB.[8] In more than 80% of cases there is spontaneous cessation of hemorrhage.[9] Although there is an absence of consensus about definitions of severity, clinicians assess severity based on hemodynamic status, laboratory findings, and associated comorbid conditions. Unlike UGIB, risk stratification for LGIB is not well defined. Velayos and colleagues[10] identified hemodynamic instability (systolic blood pressure <100 mm Hg, heart rate >100 per minute) 1 hour after initial evaluation, active gross bleeding per rectum, and an initial hematocrit of less than 35% as predictors of increased severity and poor outcomes from LGIB (79% of patients with three risk factors had recurrent or ongoing bleeding compared with 54% with two risk factors, 17% with one risk factor, and 0% with no risk factors). In another study, Strate and colleagues[11] identified heart rate greater than 100, systolic blood pressure less than 115 m Hg, syncope, nontender abdominal examination, bleeding per rectum during the first 4 hours of evaluation, history of aspirin use, and more than two active comorbid conditions as risk factors predictive of a severe course or recurrence of LGIB (patients with four or more risk factors were in the highest risk group). Das and colleagues[12] developed and externally validated an artificial neural network to predict the risk of death, rebleeding, and need for intervention in LGIB. This tool accurately predicted these outcomes and had a negative predictive value of 98% in the internal and external validation cohorts suggesting that it could be used to triage low-risk patients to outpatient management. Although artificial neural network models outperform prediction tools developed through logistic modeling, requirements for advanced software and data entry currently limit their clinical use. Use of risk stratification methods allows for triage of patients, particularly those at lower risk. Risk scoring systems for LGIB need further prospective evaluation and validation in diverse settings. Nevertheless, clinical judgment in conjunction with readily available data, such as vital signs and routine laboratory studies, is frequently sufficient to estimate severity of bleed and subsequently guide plan of care.

## ETIOLOGIES

In about 10% of cases a brisk UGI bleed presents as hematochezia and may be misdiagnosed as an LGIB.[13] In these instances bleeding is usually associated with hemodynamic instability. It is important to consider and rule out a UGI source in all patients presenting as LGIB who have associated hemodynamic instability. The presence of blood in a nasogastric tube aspirate is highly specific for a UGI source proximal to the ligament of Treitz; however, absence of a bloody return does not help exclude an UGI cause. The most common cause of LGIB is diverticular disease. Other causes include angiodysplasia, inflammatory bowel disease, postpolypectomy bleeding, neoplasia, and small bowel bleeding.[14] The causes of chronic LGIB frequently presenting as iron deficiency anemia is more difficult to discern. The causes of LGIB and their relative frequencies of occurrence are shown in **Tables 1** and **2**.

## CLINICAL PRESENTATION

In comparison with UGIB, patients with LGIB are less frequently orthostatic, have a lesser need for blood transfusion, and present with higher hemoglobin levels.[8] Although less severe than UGIB, LGIB can have a spectrum of presentation that ranges from occult to massive and life threatening. Clinical manifestations vary depending on the cause and rapidity of bleeding. Massive or rapid bleeds are usually associated with ongoing hematochezia or bright red blood per rectum; hemodynamic instability (tachycardia, hypotension, and/or syncope); and other clinical signs of shock, such as cool extremities, low urine output, and prolonged capillary refill time. Whether a patient with LGIB presents with hematochezia or melena depends on the amount of bleed and transit time. Slower bleeds, especially those occurring near the cecum, may present as melena.

**Table 1**
**Sources of hematochezia**

| Source/Finding | Frequency (%) |
|---|---|
| Diverticulum | 17–40 |
| Angiodysplasia | 9–21 |
| Colitis (ischemic, infectious, chronic inflammatory bowel disease, radiation injury) | 2–30 |
| Neoplasia, postpolypectomy bleeding | 11–14 |
| Anorectal disease (including rectal varices) | 4–10 |
| Upper gastrointestinal bleeding | 0–11 |
| Small bowel bleeding | 2–9 |

**Table 2**
**Colonic causes of iron deficiency anemia**

| Finding | Frequency (%) |
|---|---|
| Colon carcinoma | 4.5–11 |
| Angiodysplasia | 0.9–8.5 |
| Colon polyps | 2.8–7.2 |
| Colitis | 1.4–2 |
| Total colonic causes | 18–30 |

## INITIAL MANAGEMENT

The evaluation of a patient with LGIB entails a thorough history and physical examination. This should, however, not delay immediate resuscitation in an overtly bleeding patient presenting with frank or occult shock. Resuscitation strategies are discussed later in this article. Direct observation of the bloody stool is necessary to characterize the bleeding: hematochezia (frank blood, maroon stools, or blood clots) or melena. Hematochezia may be from an upper source if the bleed is brisk; conversely, melena may signal a slow right colonic or cecal bleed. History should include details about pain associated with the bleed; anticoagulant and NSAID use; comorbid conditions especially vascular disease, which may predispose to ischemic colitis; past bleeding episodes; recent colonoscopy; and symptoms suggestive of colonic malignancy. Physical examination should focus on stability of vital signs, careful abdominal examination, bowel sounds, and a digital rectal examination. The initial laboratory evaluation includes a complete blood count, coagulation profile, basic metabolic panel, and a sample for type and crossmatch.

## RESUSCITATION STRATEGIES

Patients with ongoing bleeding, significant blood loss and transfusion needs, hemodynamic instability, or high-risk features as discussed previously need to be monitored and resuscitated in an intensive care unit setting. Adequate intravenous access should be obtained (two large-bore peripheral intravenous catheters or central venous access). If massive transfusion is required, clinicians should be cognizant that large-bore peripheral catheters have larger diameters than central venous catheters and therefore resuscitation through large-bore peripheral intravenous lines may be quicker. If central venous access is required in cases of massive hemorrhage it is better to place introducer lines that have a much larger diameter than regular central venous catheters. Careful vigilance should be maintained while interpreting laboratory values; in cases of early presentation of brisk bleeds the hemoglobin and hematocrit values may not be abnormal. Physical signs of hypovolemia should be immediately recognized and rapidly corrected. The goal of resuscitation is to expediently restore effective circulating volume. Isotonic crystalloid solutions are initially used for volume replacement. Although appropriate for initial stabilization, excessive use of replacement solutions should be avoided. Blood volume replacement with PRBC should be initiated quickly if there is inadequate response to 1 to 2 L of crystalloid. If more than 3 to 4 units of PRBC are required rapidly, consideration should be given to replacement of plasma and platelets. The optimal hemoglobin targets in LGIB are controversial. In a recent study, a trigger transfusion threshold of 7 g/dL was associated with better outcomes compared with a trigger transfusion threshold of 9 g/dL in patients with UGIB who were not exsanguinating.[15] No such studies have been performed in LGIB; however, the clinical picture (rapidity of bleed, age, comorbid conditions, and hemodynamic status) should dictate transfusion thresholds and targets. For example, a higher threshold and target is probably appropriate in an elderly patient with coronary artery disease and a brisk bleed compared with a young patient without comorbidities.

Often LGIB occurs in the setting of coagulopathy or prescription of antiplatelet agents. Coagulopathy should be corrected with fresh frozen plasma and/or platelet transfusion. Transfusion of platelets may be required for antiplatelet drug use even if the platelet count is normal, because platelet function may be irreversibly inhibited. Caution should be exercised in holding the antiplatelet agent or transfusing platelets in cases where the indication for the antiplatelet agent is the presence of a stent. In these situations if the antiplatelet agent is held, it should be resumed as soon as possible. Vitamin K can be given if the coagulopathy is secondary to use of vitamin K antagonists. The onset of action even if given intravenously is, however, slower than infusion of plasma. In such cases as concomitant severe systolic dysfunction where administration of excess volume is an issue, newer products, such as prothrombin complex concentrates, can be used. These newer products may also be useful in the reversal of coagulopathy from novel anticoagulant agents, such as Factor Xa antagonists.

It should be emphasized that for brisk ongoing blood loss from LGIB, attempts to evaluate and terminate the source of bleeding should ideally proceed simultaneously, because resuscitation strategies are unlikely to be successful if the source of hemorrhage is not controlled. The method used to control source of hemorrhage (intervention via colonoscopy, angiography, or surgery) depends on the source of bleed, ability to localize, and comorbid conditions. A general management scheme is outlined in **Fig. 1**.

## COLONOSCOPY

Although many LGIBs spontaneously cease without intervention,[16,17] evaluation of the source of bleed is undertaken in most cases. Colonoscopy remains the main modality for evaluation of the source of LGIB.[18] It should be emphasized that strong consideration should be given to performance of UGI endoscopy before colonoscopy in patients presenting with hematochezia and hemodynamic instability to rule out an upper source of bleeding. The advantage of colonoscopy is that it is used for diagnostic and more importantly therapeutic purposes even in the absence of ongoing bleeding. The diagnostic yield is variable with older literature reporting rates ranging from 48% to 100%.[19] More recent literature cites rates approximating 74% to 100%.[20] The variability in rates is attributable to differences in definitions of bleeding source, patient selection criteria, and timing of colonoscopy. Affirmation that a visualized lesion is the source of hemorrhage is generally validated by an active bleed, blood clot over a visible vessel, or a clot adherent to a diverticular ulceration or the neck of a diverticulum. Just the presence of blood at a site within the colon yields little diagnostic information because of the associated intestinal peristalsis. Because of the high diagnostic yield, colonoscopy is commonly used as the initial diagnostic test in patients with LGIB who can be stabilized and undergo colon preparation.

In addition to its diagnostic capabilities, colonoscopy is also used for therapeutic purposes to achieve endoscopic hemostasis. Hemostatic techniques include thermal coagulation (electrocoagulation, argon plasma coagulation, or laser-mediated coagulation), injection therapy (epinephrine), or metallic clipping and banding.[1] In a review of published series Strate and Naumann[20] demonstrated that endoscopic therapy was

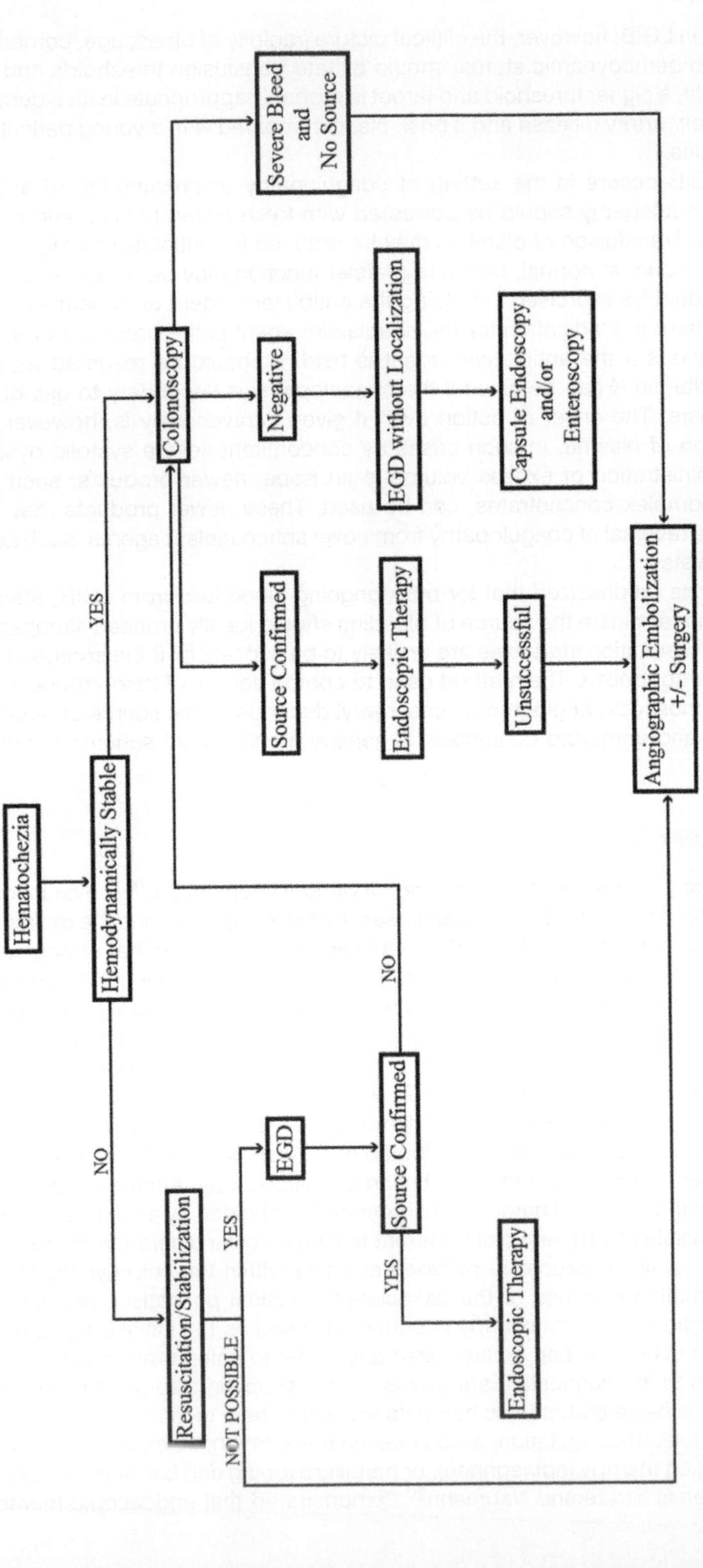


**Fig. 1.** Approach to management of a patient with lower gastrointestinal bleeding. EGD, esophagogastroduodenoscopy.

applied to 10% to 40% of patients undergoing colonoscopy for LGIB and the most commonly used modality was thermal coagulation in combination with injection therapy.

The optimal timing of colonoscopy is controversial. In a study of two sequential cohorts of severe diverticular bleeds, Jensen and colleagues[21] demonstrated that urgent colonoscopy (within 6–12 hours of admission) and subsequent endoscopic treatment reduced the rates of rebleeding and surgery compared with historical control subjects that received colonoscopy but underwent surgery if there was ongoing bleeding. In the first randomized control trial of LGIB, Green and colleagues[22] demonstrated that although a source of LGIB was identified in patients undergoing urgent colonoscopy (within 12 hours), there were no differences in rebleeding rates, transfusion requirements, mortality, or length of stay compared with the standard arm (elective colonoscopy within 74 hours). Similarly, another randomized control trial found no differences in outcomes between colonoscopy within 12 hours and colonoscopy within 36 to 60 hours.[23] Based on the available evidence, rather than a one size fits all approach, it is prudent to time colonoscopy based on the briskness of the bleed and clinical signs and symptoms. In patients with severe bleeds consideration should be given to performing colonoscopy rapidly (within 12 hours). However, it is evident from the literature that performing colonoscopy early is associated with a much better diagnostic yield.

The literature is conflicted on the issue of colon preparation before colonoscopy. Endoscopy and gastroenterology organizations advocate oral bowel preparation to improve visualization and reduce the risk of endoscopic injury.[24] Older studies reported visualization up to the cecum in only 55% to 70% of cases when colonoscopy was performed without preparation.[25] With preparation, a definitive diagnosis was obtained in 91% of patients.[20] However, Chaudhry and colleagues[26] reported a 97% diagnostic yield for emergency colonoscopy even in the absence of oral preparation. Nevertheless, performance of colonoscopy without preparation is exceedingly rare. It is feasible to administer the bowel preparation over 3 to 4 hours to facilitate early colonoscopy and this approach should be adopted especially in severe cases of LGIB.

Complications rates with even emergency colonoscopy are extremely low: 0.6% with emergency colonoscopy versus 0.3% for elective in a comprehensive review.[20] The major complication is colon perforation. Rarely volume overload, precipitation of heart failure, and electrolyte abnormalities may occur as a result of administration of bowel preparation.

## COMMON ETIOLOGIES

### *Diverticular Bleeding*

Diverticular bleeding usually presents as painless hematochezia in an older individual. Although reported to be the most common cause of LGIB (30%–50% of cases with massive LGIB),[27,28] diverticulosis is often cited as the source of bleed during colonoscopy for lack of evidence of an alternative source. Diverticulosis occurs most commonly in the left colon; however, diverticula in the right colon are more likely to bleed.[29] Bleeding is limited in about 70% to 80% of cases, however there is a high rate of recurrence. Bleeding recurs in 22% to 38% of cases after the first episode and in more than 50% of cases after the second episode.[30] Risk factors for diverticular bleeding include older age, smoking alcohol use, NSAID use, bilateral diverticulosis, hypertension, diabetes, ischemic heart disease, and obesity.[31] Risk factors for early rebleeding (within 30 days of initial treatment) include shock and active bleeding during the initial colonoscopy.[32] Because most diverticular bleeds are self-limited, evaluation with colonoscopy fails to identify an overt bleeding or stigmata of recent hemorrhage (nonbleeding visible vessel, adherent clot, or active bleeding from a diverticulum). Early colonoscopy may improve the diagnostic yield and may lead to therapeutic interventions that prevent recurrence of bleeding.[21] Once a bleeding lesion is identified it is usually amenable to endoscopic hemostasis using epinephrine injection, clipping, or thermal coagulation techniques.

### *Angiodysplasia*

Angiodysplasias are an important cause of acute and chronic LGIB. Most of these lesions are located in the right side of the colon and are often multiple in number. The number of lesions increases with advancing age. Most do not bleed or are not routinely visualized on screening colonoscopy.[33] Hence, most patients who harbor angiodysplasias are asymptomatic. Usually a precipitating factor, such as coagulopathy or NSAID use, triggers bleeding. Usually bleeding presents as painless hematochezia. On endoscopic examination angiodysplasias appear as red circumscribed lesions measuring up to a few centimeters. They are a common cause of small bowel bleeding. Bleeding usually stops spontaneously but the risk of rebleeding is high. Before ascribing bleed to these lesions, it is prudent to demonstrate active bleeding or stigmata of recent hemorrhage. Endoscopic therapies may be used to achieve hemostasis.

## OTHER MODALITIES OF DIAGNOSIS AND THERAPY

### *Radionuclide Studies*

A radionuclide scan using 99mTc-pertechnetate-labeled red blood cells can aid in localizing the bleeding site in cases where colonoscopy is not diagnostic. This is used before angiographic evaluation. This scan detects bleeding at rates of 0.1 mL/min.[34] Labeled red blood cells are stable for 48 hours; this allows for repeat imaging within that period to detect recurrent bleeding. A positive scan points to the site of bleeding in the abdomen, but is unable to localize the exact site of bleeding (**Fig. 2**). A positive scan should be used to guide further testing using either endoscopy or angiography. Patients with a positive radionuclide scan on early imaging sequences are likely to have a positive angiography.[35]

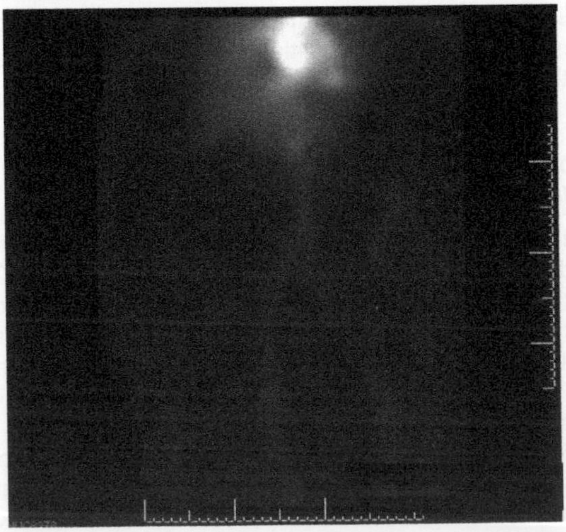

**Fig. 2.** Positive radionuclide test with abnormal radiotracer activity that appears near the splenic flexure.

### *Angiography Therapy*

Angiography can detect active bleeding when there is bleeding at a rate of at least 0.5 mL/min. Angiography is appropriate in patients with massive bleeding when colonoscopy is not possible, or in cases of recurrent bleeding after negative colonoscopy.

The diagnostic yield of angiography ranges from 40% to 78%. In cases of obscure bleeding, a radionuclide scan is usually performed first before angiography because it has a higher sensitivity and can detect bleeding at a lower rate compared with angiography. A positive radionuclide scan should be followed by angiography. Angiography has the advantage of being a diagnostic and therapeutic technique, because a bleeding site can immediately be embolized during the same procedure (**Fig. 3**). Diverticular bleeding is the most common bleeding etiology treated with angiography.

Major complications occur in 17% of patients.[20] These include bowel infarction, nephrotoxicity, hematomas, and vascular dissections. Therefore, angiography should be reserved to cases of severe bleeding in which colonoscopy is not feasible or failed to localize a bleeding source. In cases where angiography is unsuccessful at localization or therapy in a patient with massive bleeding, then emergent surgical therapy is indicated.

### *Surgical Therapy*

In patients presenting with massive LGIB in whom colonoscopic or angiographic localization and therapy has failed, surgery is indicated. Patients in whom the source of bleeding was not localized should undergo a subtotal colectomy; a more limited surgery is performed if the source of the bleeding is known (eg, right hemicolectomy for ascending colon bleeding). In patients with diffuse diverticular disease, a segmental colectomy that involves the bleeding site is adequate for therapy.

## OTHER ETIOLOGIES OF LOWER GASTROINTESTINAL BLEEDING

### *Postpolypectomy Bleeding*

Bleeding is an uncommon complication after colonoscopy and polypectomy. This occurs in 1% of cases, and commonly occurs 4 to 7 days after polypectomy, with a range

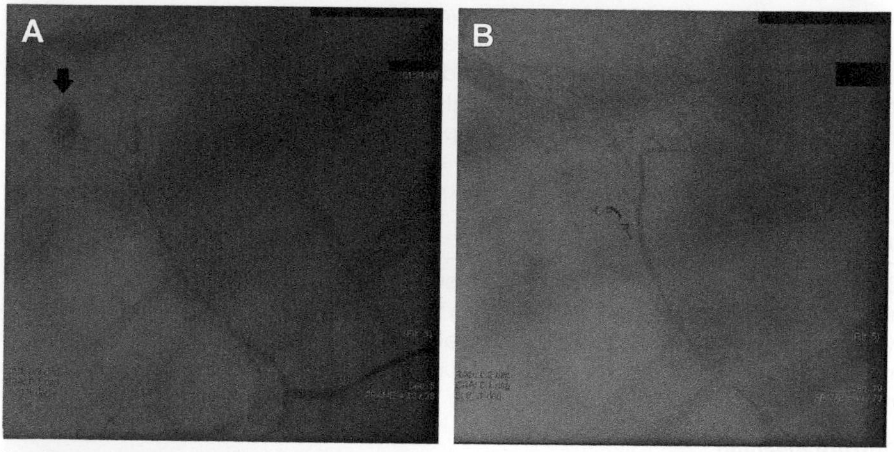


**Fig. 3.** Angiography. (*A*) Superior mesenteric angiogram with active extravasation of contrast in the area of the hepatic flexure in a patient with severe lower gastrointestinal bleeding. *Arrow* indicates active extravasation of contrast in the area of the hepatic flexure (*B*) Same patient following coil embolization.

of 1 to 14 days.[36] Risk factors for postpolypectomy bleeding include large polyp size of more than 2 cm, thick stalk, location in the right side of the colon, and use of anticoagulants (Coumadin) and antiplatelet therapy (aspirin, clopidogrel). Most cases are self-limited, and the bleeding resolves without intervention. In patients with significant bleeding, management is similar to other causes of lower GI bleeding. The patient should be resuscitated with intravenous fluids and blood transfusion, followed by a bowel preparation and colonoscopy for diagnosis and therapy. If the polyp is known to be on the left side of the colon, a simple flexible sigmoidoscopy is sufficient for examination. The site of the polypectomy is examined for stigmata of major bleeding, such as a visible or bleeding vessel. Clots should be irrigated to examine the underlying defect. Endoscopic therapy is similar to that used in upper endoscopy, and includes clip application, bipolar electrocoagulation, and epinephrine injection. In severe cases, interventional radiology and embolization maybe required to control bleeding. A clip placed during endoscopy aids in localizing the lesion during angiography. Extreme cases may require surgical resection. Prevention of postpolypectomy bleeding requires optimizing the patient's coagulation status before polypectomy. Anticoagulants should be discontinued before endoscopic polypectomy and for at least 5 days postprocedure, depending on the size of the polyp resected and the patient's thrombotic risk. Although it seems safe to resect polyps on low-dose aspirin (81 mg), all other antiplatelet agents should be discontinued before polypectomy. Before resection of large pedunculated polyps, prophylactic injection of epinephrine or the use of detachable snares reduces the risk of postpolypectomy bleeding.

### *Ischemic Colitis*

Colonic ischemic is responsible for 9% to 24% of cases of lower GI bleeding admitted to the hospital, with a mortality of 4% to 12%.[37] It could be the result of occlusive disease (arterial thrombosis or embolism, venous thrombosis), or nonocclusive ischemia as a result of cardiogenic or septic shock. Certain medications can also precipitate colonic ischemia including digoxin, alosetron, amphetamines, and cocaine abuse. Patients usually present with abdominal pain, hemodynamic instability, and moderate to severe hematochezia. Typical comorbid conditions include cardiovascular disease (congestive heart failure, atrial fibrillation, and coronary heart disease), diabetes, hypertension, chronic kidney disease, hypovolemia, or septic shock. The areas of the colon most commonly affected are the splenic flexure and the rectosigmoid junction. Right-sided colonic ischemia is associated with increased mortality compared with left-sided involvement.[38] Endoscopy reveals ulcerations, erythema, edema, and submucosal hemorrhage. However, with supportive care, most endoscopic findings resolve within a few days of the acute episode. Bleeding is usually self-limited, although ischemic colitis is associated with increased mortality.

### *Dieulafoy Lesion*

Colorectal Dieulafoy lesions are a rare cause of lower GI bleeding. This consists of an aberrant submucosal vessel that protrudes through the mucosa and is not associated with a surrounding ulcer. Bleeding is usually intermittent and severe.[39] Endoscopic treatment consists of clip placement, bipolar electrocoagulation, and epinephrine injection.

### *Obscure Bleeding*

In cases in which colonoscopy is negative for a source of bleeding, further examination of the intestinal tract is indicated. The first step is to rule out a UGI source of bleeding. This is especially important in patients with risk factors for peptic ulcer disease or those with chronic liver disease and cirrhosis. If the upper endoscopic examination does not reveal the source of bleeding, then further examination of the small bowel is required. At this point the bleeding is labeled "obscure" and because it is associated with hematochezia, it is called "obscure overt bleeding."

Lesions associated with obscure overt bleeding in this setting are most commonly found in the small intestine, with angiodysplasia being the most common in patients older than 40 years of age. Younger patients have a higher likelihood of having small intestinal tumors as a source of bleeding.

There have been several advancements in the endoscopic examination of the small intestine over the past two decades. Wireless capsule endoscopy is a noninvasive method that examines the entire length of the small intestine. It is propelled through the small bowel by peristaltic contractions. Images are sent wirelessly to a recorder and downloaded on computer for examination. Although this modality does not allow therapeutic intervention, the information obtained from this examination provides guidance for further management. If a lesion is found in the proximal small intestine, it may be amenable to examination using push enteroscopy, whereas lesions found more distally in the small intestine (beyond the proximal jejunum) can be reached using deep enteroscopy (discussed next). In the setting of obscure overt bleeding, capsule endoscopy is most useful when performed close to the bleeding episode (within 48 hours), with a high diagnostic yield of 74% to 100%.[40–42]

Push enteroscopy uses the pediatric colonoscope, which is passed transorally into the proximal small intestine. It examines the first 90 to 150 cm of the small intestine. It has a small incremental yield beyond a regular upper endoscopy, which examines the stomach and first and second part of the small intestine. The most common lesion found on this examination is angiodysplasia.

In the past decade, deep enteroscopy was introduced as a useful diagnostic and therapeutic procedure to examine the small bowel. Balloon-assisted enteroscopy is the most common technique and it involves an enteroscope with a special overtube that is equipped with one or two balloons at the distal ends of the overtube. The balloons, when inflated, act to stabilize the small bowel allowing for easier and deeper insertion of the enteroscope through the small bowel. This maneuver pleats the small intestine over the enteroscope. This procedure can be performed through the mouth (anterograde examination) or per rectum (retrograde examination). It is possible to examine the entire small bowel using this technque.[43] The diagnostic and therapeutic yield of balloon-assisted enteroscopy varies among studies but ranges between 43% and 81%.[44–46] In most cases, however, noninvasive testing of the small intestine with a wireless capsule endoscopy is performed first, and the results are used to guide further examination of the small intestine using the anterograde or retrograde examination.[47,48]

## SUMMARY

LGIB is a common clinical condition that is mostly self-limited, although severe cases can occur especially in older individuals and those on antiplatelet or anticoagulation therapy. Resuscitation principles are similar to those used in UGIB. Colonoscopy is a key diagnostic modality, although the optimal timing and the exact role in lower GI bleeding is still unclear. In practice, significant bleeding is most commonly secondary to diverticulosis and is infrequently present during colonoscopic examination. Nevertheless, colonoscopy is a therapeutic procedure because actively bleeding diverticula and other lesions (eg, arteriovenous malformations) are treated during colonoscopy. Radionuclide studies and angiography are alternative diagnostic modalities. Therapy is provided during angiography in the form of embolization, although this is associated with significant side effects. Surgery is the last resort and usually performed when there is massive bleeding that is uncontrolled using the other techniques.

## REFERENCES


1. Barnert J, Messmann H. Diagnosis and management of lower gastrointestinal bleeding [review]. Nat Rev Gastroenterol Hepatol 2009;6(11):637–46.
2. Prakash C, Zuckerman GR. Acute small bowel bleeding: a distinct entity with significantly different economic implications compared with GI bleeding from other locations. Gastrointest Endosc 2003;58(3):330–5.
3. Zuccaro G Jr. Management of the adult patient with acute lower gastrointestinal bleeding. American College of Gastroenterology. Practice Parameters Committee. Am J Gastroenterol 1998;93(8):1202–8.
4. Longstreth GF. Epidemiology and outcome of patients hospitalized with acute lower gastrointestinal hemorrhage: a population-based study. Am J Gastroenterol 1997;92(3):419–24.
5. Farrell JJ, Friedman LS. Review article: the management of lower gastrointestinal bleeding [review]. Aliment Pharmacol Ther 2005;21(11):1281–98.
6. Strate LL, Ayanian JZ, Kotler G, et al. Risk factors for mortality in lower intestinal bleeding. Clin Gastroenterol Hepatol 2008;6(9):1004–10 [quiz: 955].
7. Marion Y, Lebreton G, Le Pennec V, et al. The management of lower gastrointestinal bleeding [review]. J Visc Surg 2014;151(3):191–201.
8. Peura DA, Lanza FL, Gostout CJ, et al. The American College of Gastroenterology bleeding registry: preliminary findings. Am J Gastroenterol 1997;92(6): 924–8.
9. Zuckerman GR, Prakash C. Acute lower intestinal bleeding: part I: clinical presentation and diagnosis [review]. Gastrointest Endosc 1998;48(6):606–17.
10. Velayos FS, Williamson A, Sousa KH, et al. Early predictors of severe lower gastrointestinal bleeding and adverse outcomes: a prospective study. Clin Gastroenterol Hepatol 2004;2(6):485–90.
11. Strate LL, Saltzman JR, Ookubo R, et al. Validation of a clinical prediction rule for severe acute lower intestinal bleeding. Am J Gastroenterol 2005;100(8): 1821–7.
12. Das A, Ben-Menachem T, Cooper GS, et al. Prediction of outcome in acute lower-gastrointestinal haemorrhage based on an artificial neural network: internal and external validation of a predictive model. Lancet 2003;362(9392):1261–6.
13. Jensen DM, Machicado GA. Diagnosis and treatment of severe hematochezia. The role of urgent colonoscopy after purge. Gastroenterology 1988; 95(6):1569–74.
14. Zuckerman GR, Prakash C. Acute lower intestinal bleeding. Part II: etiology, therapy, and outcomes [review]. Gastrointest Endosc 1999;49(2):228–38.
15. Villanueva C, Colomo A, Bosch A, et al. Transfusion strategies for acute upper gastrointestinal bleeding. N Engl J Med 2013;368(1):11–21.
16. Richter JM, Christensen MR, Kaplan LM, et al. Effectiveness of current technology in the diagnosis and management of lower gastrointestinal hemorrhage. Gastrointest Endosc 1995;41(2):93–8.
17. Schmulewitz N, Fisher DA, Rockey DC. Early colonoscopy for acute lower GI bleeding predicts shorter hospital stay: a retrospective study of experience in a single center. Gastrointest Endosc 2003;58(6):841–6.

18. Eisen GM, Dominitz JA, Faigel DO, et al, American Society for Gastrointestinal Endoscopy, Standards of Practice Committee. An annotated algorithmic approach to acute lower gastrointestinal bleeding. Gastrointest Endosc 2001; 53(7):859–63.
19. Angtuaco TL, Reddy SK, Drapkin S, et al. The utility of urgent colonoscopy in the evaluation of acute lower gastrointestinal tract bleeding: a 2-year experience from a single center. Am J Gastroenterol 2001;96(6):1782–5.
20. Strate LL, Naumann CR. The role of colonoscopy and radiological procedures in the management of acute lower intestinal bleeding [review]. Clin Gastroenterol Hepatol 2010;8(4):333–43 [quiz: e44].
21. Jensen DM, Machicado GA, Jutabha R, et al. Urgent colonoscopy for the diagnosis and treatment of severe diverticular hemorrhage. N Engl J Med 2000; 342(2):78–82.
22. Green BT, Rockey DC, Portwood G, et al. Urgent colonoscopy for evaluation and management of acute lower gastrointestinal hemorrhage: a randomized controlled trial. Am J Gastroenterol 2005;100(11):2395–402.
23. Laine L, Shah A. Randomized trial of urgent vs. elective colonoscopy in patients hospitalized with lower GI bleeding. Am J Gastroenterol 2010;105(12):2636–41 [quiz: 2642].
24. Davila RE, Rajan E, Adler DG, et al, Standards of Practice Committee. ASGE Guideline: the role of endoscopy in the patient with lower-GI bleeding. Gastrointest Endosc 2005;62(5):656–60.
25. Ohyama T, Sakurai Y, Ito M, et al. Analysis of urgent colonoscopy for lower gastrointestinal tract bleeding. Digestion 2000;61(3):189–92.
26. Chaudhry V, Hyser MJ, Gracias VH, et al. Colonoscopy: the initial test for acute lower gastrointestinal bleeding. Am Surg 1998;64(8):723–8.
27. Laine L, Yang H, Chang SC, et al. Trends for incidence of hospitalization and death due to GI complications in the United States from 2001 to 2009. Am J Gastroenterol 2012;107(8):1190–5 [quiz: 1196].
28. Gayer C, Chino A, Lucas C, et al. Acute lower gastrointestinal bleeding in 1,112 patients admitted to an urban emergency medical center. Surgery 2009;146(4):600–6.
29. Wong SK, Ho YH, Leong AP, et al. Clinical behavior of complicated right-sided and left-sided diverticulosis. Dis Colon Rectum 1997;40(3):344–8.
30. McGuire HH Jr. Bleeding colonic diverticula. A reappraisal of natural history and management. Ann Surg 1994;220(5):653–6.
31. Yamada A, Sugimoto T, Kondo S, et al. Assessment of the risk factors for colonic diverticular hemorrhage. Dis Colon Rectum 2008;51(1):116–20.
32. Fujino Y, Inoue Y, Onodera M, et al. Risk factors for early re-bleeding and associated hospitalization in patients with colonic diverticular bleeding. Colorectal Dis 2013;15(8):982–6.
33. Foutch PG, Rex DK, Lieberman DA. Prevalence and natural history of colonic angiodysplasia among healthy asymptomatic people. Am J Gastroenterol 1995;90(4):564–7.
34. Thorne DA, Datz FL, Remley K, et al. Bleeding rates necessary for detecting acute gastrointestinal bleeding with technetium-99m-labeled red blood cells in an experimental model. J Nucl Med 1987;28(4):514–20.
35. Ng DA, Opelka FG, Beck DE, et al. Predictive value of technetium Tc 99m-labeled red blood cell scintigraphy for positive angiogram in massive lower gastrointestinal hemorrhage. Dis Colon Rectum 1997;40(4):471–7.
36. Zuccaro G. Epidemiology of lower gastrointestinal bleeding. Best Pract Res Clin Gastroenterol 2008;22(2):225–32.

37. Brandt LJ, Feuerstadt P, Longstreth GF, et al. ACG clinical guideline: epidemiology, risk factors, patterns of presentation, diagnosis, and management of colon ischemia (CI). Am J Gastroenterol 2015;110(1):18–44.
38. Brandt LJ, Feuerstadt P, Blaszka MC. Anatomic patterns, patient characteristics, and clinical outcomes in ischemic colitis: a study of 313 cases supported by histology. Am J Gastroenterol 2010;105(10):2245–52.
39. Lee YK, Bair MJ, Chen HL, et al. A case of massive lower gastrointestinal bleeding from a rectal Dieulafoy lesion. Advances in Digestive Medicine; 2(3):108–10.
40. Goenka MK, Majumder S, Kumar S, et al. Single center experience of capsule endoscopy in patients with obscure gastrointestinal bleeding. World J Gastroenterol 2011;17(6):774–8.
41. Yamada A, Watabe H, Kobayashi Y, et al. Timing of capsule endoscopy influences the diagnosis and outcome in obscure-overt gastrointestinal bleeding. Hepatogastroenterology 2012;59(115):676–9.
42. Hartmann D, Schmidt H, Bolz G, et al. A prospective two-center study comparing wireless capsule endoscopy with intraoperative enteroscopy in patients with obscure GI bleeding. Gastrointest Endosc 2005;61(7):826–32.
43. Fisher L, Lee Krinsky M, Anderson MA, et al. The role of endoscopy in the management of obscure GI bleeding. Gastrointest Endosc 2010;72(3):471–9.
44. Foutch PG, Sawyer R, Sanowski RA. Push-enteroscopy for diagnosis of patients with gastrointestinal bleeding of obscure origin. Gastrointest Endosc 1990;36(4): 337–41.
45. Triester SL, Leighton JA, Leontiadis GI, et al. A meta-analysis of the yield of capsule endoscopy compared to other diagnostic modalities in patients with obscure gastrointestinal bleeding. Am J Gastroenterol 2005;100(11):2407–18.
46. Rex DK, Lappas JC, Maglinte DD, et al. Enteroclysis in the evaluation of suspected small intestinal bleeding. Gastroenterology 1989;97(1):58–60.
47. DiSario JA, Petersen BT, Tierney WM, et al. Enteroscopes. Gastrointest Endosc 2007;66(5):872–80.
48. Shabana FP, Jonathan AL, Ananya D, et al. Double-balloon enteroscopy and capsule endoscopy have comparable diagnostic yield in small-bowel disease: a meta-analysis. Clin Gastroenterol Hepatol 2008;6(6):671–6.

# Role of the Open Abdomen in Critically Ill Patients

Marshall Beckman, MD, Jasmeet Paul, MD, Todd Neideen, MD, John A. Weigelt, MD, DVM*

**KEYWORDS**

- Open abdomen • Abdominal compartment syndrome
- Temporary abdominal closure • Negative pressure wound therapy
- Retroperitoneal Hemorrhage • Intra-abdominal infections • Damage control surgery

**KEY POINTS**

- An open abdomen is commonly used in critically ill patients to temporize permanent abdominal closure for clinical reasons.
- The most common reason for leaving the abdomen open by reopening a laparotomy, not closing, or creating a fresh laparotomy is the abdominal compartment syndrome.
- The open abdomen technique is also used in damage control operations and intra-abdominal sepsis.
- Negative pressure wound therapy may be associated with better outcomes than other temporary abdominal closure techniques.
- The open abdomen is associated with many early and late complications, including infections, gastrointestinal fistulas, and ventral hernias. Clinicians should be vigilant regarding the development of these complications.

An open abdomen is defined as purposely foregoing fascial closure of the abdomen after the cavity is opened. It is most commonly used after a midline laparotomy or celiotomy. The goal is to temporize abdominal closure for a clinical reason and return in a short period of time to effect complete fascial closure. While the abdomen is open, the patient's disease or condition is stabilized or preferably improved. The patient is returned to the operating room and complete fascial closure is achieved under semi-elective conditions.[1]

The technique was first used by Ogilvie to treat intra-abdominal sepsis more than 75 years ago.[2] His initial intent was to leave the abdomen open, allowing the intra-abdominal infection to drain like any other infected wound, which would achieve the

Disclosures: None.
Division of Trauma Surgery and Critical Care, Department of Surgery, Medical College of Wisconsin, 9200 West Wisconsin Avenue, Milwaukee, WI 53226, USA
* Corresponding author.
*E-mail address:* jweigelt@mcw.edu

Crit Care Clin 32 (2016) 255–264
http://dx.doi.org/10.1016/j.ccc.2015.12.003 criticalcare.theclinics.com
0749-0704/16/$ – see front matter 

principle of source control.[3] Vaseline-impregnated gauze was used to protect the exposed bowel. The infection was treated, it was hoped that the patient improved, and then fascial closure was achieved 1 to 4 days later. An open abdomen continues to be used for severe peritonitis usually complicated by septic shock, but it is most commonly used as treatment of intra-abdominal hypertension causing the abdominal compartment syndrome (ACS).

## ABDOMINAL COMPARTMENT SYNDROME

One of the most common indications for not closing or reopening a laparotomy incision is the ACS. ACS represents abdominal hypertension that produces organ dysfunction secondary to the increased intra-abdominal pressure. Intra-abdominal hypertension (IAH) is defined as a bladder pressure greater than 12 to 15 mm Hg in adults. When IAH reaches 20 to 25 mm Hg and organ dysfunction is recognized, ACS is considered to be present. These pressures are relative but have been identified by the World Society of the Abdominal Compartment Syndrome.[4] The causes of IAH are considered primary or secondary. Primary IAH/ACS is associated with intraperitoneal or retroperitoneal processes such as bleeding or infection. Secondary IAH/ACS is associated with extra-abdominal processes such as bowel edema precipitated by massive fluid resuscitation of shock, which causes bowel edema or intraperitoneal fluid accumulation. Differentiation of the two types is important because the treatment steps are different.[4]

The organ dysfunction with ACS is usually recognized by changes in lung and renal function. Pulmonary dynamics change as ACS develops. Tidal volumes decrease or, if mechanical ventilation is being used, an increase in peak pressure is noted with similar tidal volumes. This process occurs as the IAH pushes the diaphragm up, decreasing the intrathoracic volume. The increased peak pressures increase the chances of barotrauma and possibly cause acute lung injury. Renal dysfunction is reflected by a decreasing urine output caused by decreased renal perfusion as the renal vein is compressed from the increased abdominal pressure. Renal blood flow is decreased as renal vascular resistance increases. Other organs that can manifest changes with ACS include cardiac and cerebral organs. As IAH increases, venous return is reduced, which causes a decrease in cardiac output despite what appear to be increased intravascular pressures. Cerebral changes are possible when the intrathoracic pressures reduce venous return from the brain. Intracranial pressure increases, which may result in cerebral edema. IAH and the ACS can produce changes in other intra-abdominal organs.[5] The bowel mucosa becomes ischemic and, after release of the IAH, a reperfusion injury can occur. Abnormal hepatic metabolism is also observed.

## DIAGNOSIS OF ABDOMINAL COMPARTMENT SYNDROME

When ACS is suspected, bladder pressures can be measured. This measurement is commonly accomplished by instilling a small amount of sterile saline into the bladder and attaching the Foley to a pressure transducer. The symphysis pubis is used as the zero point. A grading system is used for the pressure measurements. Grade I is 12 to 15 mm Hg; grade II is 16 to 20 mm Hg; grade III is 21 to 25 mm Hg; and grade IV is greater than 25 mm Hg.[6–8] Although a single bladder pressure is commonly used to detect and grade IAH, a calculation of an abdominal perfusion pressure (APP; mean arterial pressure – intra-abdominal pressure) is suggested as a better method to detect ACS. An APP greater than 60 mm Hg is suggested as an adequate goal for resuscitation when IAH is present, although this value has not been subjected to prospective trials.[9] Although abnormal physiology can be detected at all levels of IAH, grade III and IV are usually associated with organ dysfunction that is consistent with ACS and treatment steps should be instituted. Medical interventions include sedating to improve abdominal wall compliance, placing a nasogastric tube for gastric drainage, removing intraperitoneal fluid collections if present, limiting intravenous fluids if possible, diuresis, and allowing hypercarbia by reducing tidal volumes. Although all these interventions are possible, the only solution for ACS is decreasing the pressure by decompressive laparotomy.[4]

## MANAGEMENT OF THE OPEN ABDOMEN

A temporary dressing is used whenever the open abdominal technique is applied. Numerous devices are available for this dressing.[10–15] Historically, the Bogota bag was one of the first techniques. A sterile saline bag was used to cover the intra-abdominal contents by suturing to the fascial edges.[16]

There have been many developments in managing the open abdomen since the Bogota bag. There are now commercially available devices that allow tension to be placed on the fascial edges, including the Wittmann patch.[17] The commercially available devices include many that try to achieve dynamic closure as well as the negative pressure wound suction devices.[18–20] At present, the negative pressure devices seem to be favored, especially because they allow fluid collection into a designated canister and can facilitate fluid loss measurements. These dressings should be changed in the operating room or in the intensive care unit every 2 to 3 days. If the patient is not on antibiotics for other reasons, they are not necessary when using these devices.

The different approaches to management of the open abdomen have shown mixed results. Data suggest that negative pressure wound therapy may be associated with better outcomes compared with other temporary abdominal closure techniques.[21,22]

Once the temporary abdominal closure is in place, careful monitoring of the closure is needed to ensure that there is no impending evisceration. Patients who are otherwise hemodynamically normal can be extubated and sent to the ward with no sedation and the usual postoperative pain control regimen. The patient should be monitored closely for fluid balance because patients with an open abdomen have increased insensible fluid loss. A daily weight is recommended that allows careful documentation of potential fluid loss. A negative pressure wound device helps decrease evaporative losses and allows accurate measurement of fluid loss through the wound.[23] These fluid losses may or may not need to be replaced based on the overall fluid status of the patient. An isotonic solution is commonly used for replacement. As with any critically ill patient, it is important to consider management of nutrition and electrolytes.

## CAUSES OF ABDOMINAL COMPARTMENT SYNDROME

Secondary abdominal ACS is found in many clinical scenarios. Large-volume fluid resuscitation is one of the most common reasons. In blunt trauma, the incidence of ACS goes from 0.6% if less than 10 L of crystalloid are given, to 4.3% if 10 to 15 L are given, to 12.1% if more than 15 L of crystalloid are given.[24] Severe pancreatitis necessitates large-volume resuscitation to maintain an adequate circulating blood volume. Fluid accumulation in the retroperitoneum around the inflamed pancreas causes IAH and ACS.[25] Sepsis with shock can also result in bowel edema and intraperitoneal fluid accumulation, causing a similar IAH and ACS.[26] Patients with 70% total body surface area burn or greater are at risk to develop a secondary ACS as fluid resuscitation proceeds.[27]

Hemorrhagic shock can lead to IAH and ACS by a primary or secondary mechanism or both. A primary cause is hemorrhage into the abdomen or retroperitoneum directly increasing intra-abdominal pressure. A secondary cause is again resuscitation secondary to an extra-abdominal source of massive blood loss or delayed treatment of hemorrhagic shock, which increases the amount of resuscitation needed to restore normal tissue perfusion.[28–30]

A classic cause of primary IAH and ACS is a retroperitoneal bleed from a ruptured abdominal aortic aneurysm (AAA).[31] This situation is a surgical emergency and usually required a laparotomy to repair the aorta. After repair, secondary to the retroperitoneal blood and fluid resuscitation, IAH and ACS developed, forcing a reopening of the laparotomy. Endovascular repair is now more commonly used, avoiding a laparotomy. However, some of these patients develop IAH and ACS, which require a decompressive laparotomy after the aorta is successfully repaired.[32,33] Other causes of retroperitoneal bleeding can lead to ACS. A retroperitoneal bleed from anticoagulants or spontaneous hemorrhage, possibly from an adrenal source, is possible.[34]

A different indication for using an open abdomen technique is a damage control operation.[35] Damage control operation is a term used to describe an abdominal procedure in which the abdominal incision is not closed after severe bleeding and bowel contamination is controlled. These patients usually have hemorrhagic shock and require massive blood and crystalloid infusions during resuscitation. The source of bleeding is controlled, which can even include packing parts of the abdomen. Bowel injuries are repaired, usually by bowel resections, but no anastomosis is attempted secondary to the profound shock. These patients are usually cold, acidotic, and coagulopathic: the lethal triad.[36] Avoiding further surgery is desirable and the operation is truncated by packing the abdomen and placing a temporary closure device.[37,38] The patient's resuscitation is continued postoperatively in an intensive care unit. A successful resuscitation corrects the lethal triad and the patient is returned to the operating room for removal of packing, bowel anastomoses if necessary, and abdominal closure 1 to 3 days later. It is important to remember that IAH and ACS can develop in patients with temporary abdominal closure.[39] In these patients, the temporary closure is released as signs of ACS are detected.

Intra-abdominal sepsis is the last major condition that occasionally requires the use of the open abdomen technique. Perforated hollow viscus is the leading cause of intra-abdominal sepsis.[40] As mentioned earlier, Ogilvie was the first to describe the open abdomen for the treatment of severe intra-abdominal sepsis.[2] Leaving the abdomen open to treat severe peritonitis is possible, although not recommended, because repeated explorations increase the chances of a bowel injury and eventual intestinal fistula.[41,42] The goal of treating intra-abdominal sepsis is to identify and repair the perforation. A bowel resection is often necessary, especially if the diagnosis was delayed. The abdomen may be left open to allow a second-look operation to inspect the anastomosis or bowel repair. Alternatively, the abdomen is left open secondary to the resuscitation and severe bowel edema that can occur. This approach is an attempt to prevent IAH and ACS. The surgeon recognizes this potential complication as closure is attempted and inspiratory pressures begin to increase as closure commences. Communication between the surgeon and anesthesiologists is essential to recognize this potential ACS and prevent it by applying the open abdomen technique of a temporary abdominal closure.

## COMPLICATIONS OF THE OPEN ABDOMEN TECHNIQUE

There are multiple complications from the open abdomen.[43] They include mechanical and infectious complications, which occur early, and ventral herniation, which is a late complication.

## EARLY COMPLICATIONS

### *Wound Management*

The temporary dressing used to keep the intra-abdominal contents from eviscerating can fail. Minor failures are observed as leakage from the edge of the dressing requiring bolstering the dressing with tape or other occlusive materials. Major dressing failure is complete evisceration of the bowel, which requires a reapplication of the entire dressing and possibly a different dressing altogether. Other causes for the failure must always be sought. These causes can include ongoing abdominal hemorrhage, poor patient sedation, and inadequate dressing placement initially.

### *Surgical Site Infections*

Wound infections are common after the open abdomen, although the rate is confounded based on overall management of the wound. Lower rates are reported when the skin is not closed compared with reports of skin closure at the time of fascial closure.[44] There is no question that wound colonization occurs while the abdomen is open. Rasilainen and colleagues[45] studied the time course and microbiology of bacterial colonization of the open abdomen. They examined 111 consecutive patients with an open abdomen for nontrauma indications, including ACS, severe pancreatitis, open AAA repair, and peritonitis. The open abdomens were managed with a polypropylene mesh and negative pressure wound therapy (NPWT). At closure the mesh was removed and the fascia was closed primarily. Microbiologic cultures were taken of the abdomen and deep peritoneal space at each take-back and final closure. Seventy-eight percent of patients had at least 1 positive culture and most grew multiple organisms. The organisms isolated were primarily enteric gram-negative bacilli and gram-positives from the skin. The median time to colonization was 2 days and the longer the patient was treated with an open abdomen the higher the rate of colonization. No statistically significant difference was noted in primary fascial closure, fascial dehiscence, enteric fistula, surgical site infection, or intra-abdominal abscess (IA) in the patients who were colonized versus those with a sterile abdomen. These data suggest that early abdominal closure is a goal of the open abdomen technique.

After fascial closure, surgical site infection is prevented by leaving the skin open. A delayed primary closure can be attempted, but most commonly the wound is left to heal by secondary intention. Sometimes loose approximation of the skin is used so there is less of a gap for the skin cells to migrate across. Most clinicians do not advocate skin closure of any kind after intra-abdominal sepsis with an open abdomen because this increases the rate of surgical site infection.

### *Intra-Abdominal Infection*

IA is a well-described complication of the open abdomen technique. A report on patients with trauma treated with an open abdomen revealed an IA rate of 20% and a gastrointestinal fistula rate of 5%.[46] These rates may be higher if the indication of the open abdomen is intra-abdominal sepsis. The fistula can be either an enterocutaneous or enteroatmospheric type. The former occurs when the fistula exits via the skin, whereas the latter is present when the intestinal fistula exits directly to the atmosphere. These two complications can occur independently or together. A very common sequence is drainage of an IA, the cultures grow enteric contents, and a fistula eventual becomes obvious.

The initial retrospective reports on damage control laparotomy with an open abdomen had a range of IA from 7% to 20%.[44,47,48] However, infections were not the primary focus of these articles and several of them grouped IA with enterocutaneous fistula (ECF). The exact incidence of ECF is not clear but it is approximately 5% in well-done prospective studies.[41,46] The American Association for the Surgery of Trauma trial by Dubose and colleagues[46] reported a 20% incidence of IA after closure, which is similar to both Western Trauma Associations studies[4,6,41,49] and the trial by Pommerening and colleagues.[47] The rate of IA after primary fascial closure of an open abdomen is probably 20%. There may be an increase in IA rates in patients with nontrauma indications for open abdomen but in well-done prospective studies the rates seem similar, likely because of colonization of the abdomen during the take-back procedures.[45]

Management of patients who develop IA after primary fascial closure is similar to management of those who have IAA from other causes. Numerous reports show the safety and efficacy of radiology-guided percutaneous drainage with acceptable success rates.[40,50,51] There are few absolute contraindications to percutaneous drainage of an IA. Relative contraindications exist and include a significant coagulopathy that cannot be corrected, lack of a safe access window for catheter placement, and an uncooperative patient.[52] Success rates of greater than 80% are common. Failure occurs most commonly with pancreatic and postoperative collections, especially if yeast is present.[53]

### *Gastrointestinal Fistula*

An enteroatmospheric fistula is the worst complication of the open abdomen aside from death and it is one of the most challenging. Any damage to the bowel can lead to a fistula. This fistula can occur inadvertently at any time during staged abdominal closure or from the original operation. Anastomotic leak can also lead to a fistula. Suction from a vacuum closure device can erode into the bowel causing a leak. Although iatrogenic injuries during abdominal exploration can cause these fistulas, even with the best care a gastrointestinal fistula is possible when using an open abdominal approach.

Various strategies are used with an open abdomen to increase the rate of primary fascial closure and to decrease the incidence of IA and ECF. The use of NPWT[54,55] and early abdominal closure are the two techniques advocated to reduce both of these complications. Early closure is the single best approach to reduce the rate of ECF, but there is no impact on IA rates.[1] NPWT assists fascial closure by managing intra-abdominal fluid and reducing or minimizing contamination of the wound.[56] However, another report had a high rate of bacterial contamination despite application of NPWT.[57]

## LATE COMPLICATIONS

### *Ventral Hernia*

The most common late complication of an open abdomen is a ventral hernia. Ten percent of people who have definitive closure after an open abdomen develop a ventral hernia by 21 months.[58] These hernias can develop as a result of infection, fascial necrosis, or loss of domain as the abdominal muscles contract away from their normal medial position. Fascial necrosis after closure commonly occurs when attempts to close the abdomen result in excessive tension on the midline fascia causing the fascia to become ischemia. Necrosis follows and either dehiscence or evisceration occurs. If another closure is attempted, then further fascial damage can occur. The longer the abdomen is open the more difficult closure becomes. The muscles of the abdomen tend to retract when the abdomen is open because of the loss of medial tension. If they retract far enough, closure is sometimes not possible and a mesh closure with a prosthetic material is necessary. This mesh can be resorbable or permanent. Regardless, this leads to a ventral hernia.

## SUMMARY

The open abdomen continues to find new uses. It continues to be used for intra-abdominal infection, but it is useful in critically ill patients who develop the ACS from either primary or secondary causes. Understanding when it is useful and how it is managed is imperative for its proper use.

## REFERENCES

1. Demetrios D, Ali S. Management of the open abdomen. Surg Clin North Am 2014;94(1):131–53.
2. Kreis BE, de Mol van Otterloo AJ, Kreis RW. Open abdomen management: a review of its history and a proposed management algorithm. Med Sci Monit 2013;19:524–33.
3. Solomkin JS, Mazuski JE, Rodvold KA, et al. Diagnosis and management of complicated intra-abdominal infection in adults and children: guidelines by the Surgical Infection Society and the Infectious Diseases Society of America. Clin Infect Dis 2010;50(2):133–64.
4. Kirkpatrick AW, Roberts DJ, De Waele K, et al. Intra-abdominal hypertension and the abdominal compartment syndrome: updated consensus definitions and clinical practice guidelines from the World Society of the Abdominal Compartment Syndrome. Intensive Care Med 2013;39:1190–206.
5. Papavramidis TS, Marinis AD, Pliakos I, et al. Abdominal compartment syndrome – intra-abdominal hypertension: defining, diagnosing, and managing. J Emerg Trauma Shock 2011;4(2):279–91.
6. Burch JM, Moore EE, Moore FA, et al. The abdominal compartment syndrome. Surg Clin North Am 1996;76(4):833–42.
7. Malbrain M, Cheatham M, Kirkpatrick A, et al. Results from the international conference of experts on intra-abdominal hypertension and abdominal compartment syndrome, I: definitions. Intensive Care Med 2006;32(11):1722–32.
8. Lee RK. Intra-abdominal hypertension and abdominal compartment syndrome: a comprehensive overview. Crit Care Nurse 2012;32(1):19–31.
9. Cheatham ML, Malbrain MLNG. Abdominal perfusion pressure. In: Ivatury RR, Cheatham ML, Malbrain MLNG, et al, editors. Abdominal compartment syndrome. Austin (TX): Landes Biomedical; 2006. p. 69–81.
10. Wittmann DH, Aprahamian C, Bergstein JM. Etappenlavage: advanced diffuse peritonitis managed by planned multiple laparotomies utilizing zippers, slide fastener, and Velcro analogue for temporary abdominal closure. World J Surg 1990;14(2):218–26.
11. Howdieshell TR, Proctor CD, Sternberg E, et al. Temporary abdominal closure followed by definitive abdominal wall reconstruction of the open abdomen. Am J Surg 2004;188:301–6.
12. Fernandez L, Norwood S, Roettger R, et al. Temporary intravenous bag silo closure in severe abdominal trauma. J Trauma 1996;40(2):258–60.
13. Bruhin A, Ferreira F, Chariker M, et al. Systematic review and evidence based recommendations for the use of negative pressure wound therapy in the open abdomen. Int J Surg 2014;12(10):1105–14.
14. Jenkins SD, Klamer TW, Parteka JJ, et al. A comparison of prosthetic materials used to repair abdominal wall defects. Surgery 1983;94(2):392–8.

15. Lamb JP, Vitale T, Kaminski DL. Comparative evaluation of synthetic meshes used for abdominal wall replacement. Surgery 1983;93(5):643–8.
16. Kirshtein B, Roy-Shapiro A, Kantsberg L, et al. Use of the "Bogota bag" for temporary abdominal closure in patients with secondary peritonitis. Am Surg 2007; 73(3):249–52.
17. Star surgical. Burlington (WI). Available at: http://www.starsurgical.com/wp.html. Accessed September 29, 2015.
18. Fitzgerald JE, Gupta S, Masterson S, et al. Laparostomy management using the ABThera™ open abdomen negative pressure therapy system in a grade IV open abdomen secondary to acute pancreatitis. Int Wound J 2013;10(2):138–44.
19. Verdam FJ, Dolmans DE, Loos MJ, et al. Delayed primary closure of the septic open abdomen with a dynamic closure system. World J Surg 2011;35:2348.
20. Haddock C, Konkin DE, Blair NP. Management of the open abdomen with the abdominal reapproximation anchor dynamic fascial closure system. Am J Surg 2013;205:528.
21. Garner GB, Ware DN, Cocanour CS, et al. Vacuum-assisted wound closure provides early fascial reapproximation in trauma patients with open abdomens. Am J Surg 2001;182(6):630–8.
22. Roberts DJ, Zygun DA, Grendar J, et al. Negative-pressure wound therapy for critically ill adults with open abdominal wounds: a systematic review. J Trauma Acute Care Surg 2012;73:629–39.
23. Caro A, Olona C, Jiménez A, et al. Treatment of the open abdomen with topical negative pressure therapy: a retrospective study of 46 cases. Int Wound J 2011;8:274–9.
24. Kasotakis G, Sideris A, Yang Y, et al, Inflammation and Host Response to Injury Investigators. Aggressive early crystalloid resuscitation adversely affects outcomes in adult blunt trauma patients: an analysis of the glue grant database. J Trauma Acute Care Surg 2013;74(5):1215–22.
25. De Waele JJ. Management of abdominal compartment syndrome in acute pancreatitis. Pancreapedia: Exocrine Pancreas Knowledge Base 2015;1:7. Version 1.0. Available at: http://www.pancreapedia.org/reviews/management-of-abdominal-compartment-syndrome-in-acute-pancreatitis.
26. Ball CG, Kirkpatrick AW, McBeth P. The secondary abdominal compartment syndrome: not just another post-traumatic complication. Can J Surg 2008;51(5): 399–405.
27. Hobson KG, Young KM, Ciraulo A, et al. Release of abdominal compartment syndrome improves survival in patients with burn injury. J Trauma 2002;53:1129–34.
28. Balogh Z, Moore FA, Moore EE, et al. Secondary abdominal compartment syndrome: a potential threat for all trauma clinicians. Injury 2007;38:272–9.
29. Balogh Z, McKinley BA, Cocanour CS, et al. Secondary abdominal compartment syndrome is an elusive early complication of traumatic shock resuscitation. Am J Surg 2002;184:538–43.
30. Rizoli S, Mamtani A, Scarpelini S, et al. Abdominal compartment syndrome in trauma resuscitation. Curr Opin Anaesthesiol 2010;23(2):251–7.
31. Rubenstein C, Bietz G, Davenport DL, et al. Abdominal compartment syndrome associated with endovascular and open repair of ruptured abdominal aortic aneurysms. J Vasc Surg 2015;61(3):648–54.
32. Karkos CD, Menexes GC, Patelis N, et al. A systematic review and meta-analysis of abdominal compartment syndrome after endovascular repair of ruptured abdominal aortic aneurysms. J Vasc Surg 2014;59:829.

33. Djavani Gidlund K, Wanhainen A, Björck M. Intra-abdominal hypertension and abdominal compartment syndrome after endovascular repair of ruptured abdominal aortic aneurysm. Eur J Vasc Endovasc Surg 2011;41:742.
34. Dabney A, Bastani B. Enoxaparin-associated severe retroperitoneal bleeding and abdominal compartment syndrome: a report of two cases. Intensive Care Med 2001;27:1954–7.
35. Rotondo MF, Schwab CW, McGonigal MD, et al. Damage control: an approach for improved survival in exsanguinating penetrating abdominal injury. J Trauma 1993;35:375–82.
36. Hsu JM, Pham TN. Damage control in the injured patient. Int J Crit Illn Inj Sci 2011;1(1):66–72.
37. Rotondo MF, Zonies DH. The damage control sequence and underlying logic. Surg Clin North Am 1997;77:761–77.
38. Moore EE, Burch JM, Franciose RJ, et al. Staged physiologic restoration and damage control surgery. World J Surg 1998;22:1184–90.
39. Ouellet JF, Ball CG. Recurrent abdominal compartment syndrome induced by high negative pressure abdominal closure dressing. J Trauma 2011;71: 785–6.
40. Lopez N, Kobayashi L, Coimbra R. A comprehensive review of abdominal infections. World J Emerg Surg 2011;6:7.
41. Burlew CC, Moore EE, Cuschieri J, et al. Sew it up! A Western Trauma Association multi-institutional study of enteric injury management in the post injury open abdomen. J Trauma 2011;70:273.
42. Bradley MJ, Dubose JJ, Scalea TM, et al. Independent predictors of enteric fistula and abdominal sepsis after damage control laparotomy: results from the prospective AAST open abdomen registry. JAMA Surg 2013;148:947.
43. Kritayakirana K, Maggio PM, Brundage S, et al. Outcomes and complications of open abdomen technique for managing non-trauma patients. J Emerg Trauma Shock 2010;3(2):118–22.
44. Miller RS, Morris JA Jr, Diaz JJ Jr, et al. Complications after 344 damage-control open celiotomies. J Trauma 2005;59(6):1365–71.
45. Rasilainen SK, Juhani MP, Kalevi LA. Microbial colonization of open abdomen in critically ill surgical patients. World J Emerg Surg 2015;10(25):2–8.
46. DuBose JJ, Scalea TM, Holcomb JB, et al. Open abdominal management after damage-control laparotomy for trauma: a prospective observational American Association for the Surgery of Trauma multicenter study. J Trauma Acute Care Surg 2012;74(1):113–22.
47. Pommerening MJ, DuBose JJ, Zielinski MD, et al. Time to first take-back operation predicts successful primary fascial closure in patients undergoing damage control laparotomy. Surgery 2014;156(2):431–8.
48. Tsuei BJ, Skinner JC, Bernard AC, et al. The open peritoneal cavity: etiology correlates with the likelihood of fascial closure. Am Surg 2004;70(7):652–6.
49. Burlew CC, Moore EE, Cuschieri J, et al. Who should we feed? Western Trauma Association multi-institutional study of enteral nutrition in the open abdomen after injury. J Trauma Acute Care Surg 2012;73(6):1380–7.
50. Kassi F, Dohan A, Soyer P, et al. Predictive factors for failure of percutaneous drainage of postoperative abscess after abdominal surgery. Am J Surg 2014; 207(6):915–21.
51. Robert B, Yzet T, Regimbeau JM. Radiologic drainage of post-operative collections and abscesses. J Visc Surg 2013;150(3 Suppl):S11–8.

52. Wallace MJ, Chin KW, Fletcher TB, et al. Quality improvement guidelines for percutaneous drainage/aspiration of abscess and fluid collections. J Vasc Interv Radiol 2010;21:431–5.
53. Cinat ME, Wilson SE, Din AM. Determinants for successful percutaneous image-guided drainage of intra-abdominal abscess. Arch Surg 2002;137(7):845–9.
54. Acosta S, Bjarnason T, Petersson U, et al. Multicentre prospective study of fascial closure rate after open abdomen with vacuum and mesh-mediated fascial traction. Br J Surg 2011;98(5):735–43.
55. Rasilainen SK, Mentula PJ, Leppaniemi AK. Vacuum and mesh-mediated fascial traction for primary closure of the open abdomen in critically ill surgical patients. Br J Surg 2012;99(12):1725–32.
56. Bovill E, Banwell PE, Teot L, et al. Topical negative pressure wound therapy: a review of its role and guidelines for its use in the management of acute wounds. Int Wound J 2008;5(4):511–29.
57. Pliakos I, Michalopoulos N, Papavramidis TS, et al. The effect of vacuum-assisted closure in bacterial clearance of the infected abdomen. Surg Infect (Larchmt) 2014;15(1):18–23.
58. Frazee RC, Abernathy S, Jupiter D, et al. Long-term consequences of open abdomen management. Trauma 2013;16(1):37–40.

# Abdominal Circulatory Interactions

Gaurav Dagar, MD[a], Amit Taneja, MD[a], Rahul S. Nanchal, MD, MS[b,*]

**KEYWORDS**

- Mechanical ventilation • Ascites • Prone positioning • Vascular waterfall
- Abdominal zone conditions

**KEY POINTS**

- Ventilation whether spontaneous or mechanical affects abdominal pressure (Pab) by inducing diaphragmatic descent.
- Changes in Pab affect circulatory physiology through effects on venous return, preload, and LV and RV performance.
- Transmission of increased abdominal pressure to the thorax and cardiac chambers can make interpretation of static pressure in the cardiac chambers difficult.
- Changes in abdominal pressure may play a large role in common clinical conditions, such as weaning-induced cardiac dysfunction, postparacentesis circulatory dysfunction, prone positioning during ARDS, and laparoscopic surgery.
- Intensivists should have a fundamental understanding of the effects of abdominal pressure on circulatory and respiratory physiology.

The abdominal compartment is separated from the thoracic compartment by the diaphragm. Under normal circumstances, a large portion of the venous return crosses the splanchnic and nonsplanchnic abdominal regions before entering the thorax and the right side of the heart. Moreover, mechanical ventilation especially with positive end-expiratory pressure (PEEP) may affect abdominal venous return independent of its interactions at the thoracic level. Furthermore, changes in pressure in the intra-abdominal compartment may have important implications for organ function within the thorax, particularly if there is a sustained rise in intra-abdominal pressure as in abdominal compartment syndrome. It is therefore important to understand the consequences of abdominal pressure (Pab) changes on respiratory and circulatory

Disclosures: None.

[a] Division of Pulmonary and Critical Care Medicine, Medical College of Wisconsin, Suite E 5200, 9200 West Wisconsin Avenue, Milwaukee, WI 53226, USA; [b] Critical Care Fellowship Program, Medical Intensive Care Unit, Division of Pulmonary and Critical Care Medicine, Suite E 5200, 9200 West Wisconsin Avenue, Milwaukee, WI 53226, USA
* Corresponding author.
*E-mail address:* Rnanchal@mcw.edu

Crit Care Clin 32 (2016) 265–277
http://dx.doi.org/10.1016/j.ccc.2015.12.005 criticalcare.theclinics.com

physiology. This article elucidates important abdominal-respiratory-circulatory interactions and their clinical effects. The effect of intra-abdominal hypertension on systemic physiology is not a focus of this review. For a detailed discussion of this topic please see Sarani, Maluso, Olson: Abdominal Compartment Hypertension and Abdominal Compartment Syndrome, in this issue.

## RELATIONSHIP BETWEEN RIGHT ATRIAL PRESSURE, ABDOMINAL PRESSURE, AND VENOUS RETURN

Traditionally, changes in intrathoracic pressure have been the sole focus of analyses of cyclic respiratory changes in venous return. It is generally assumed that spontaneous inspiration (negative intrathoracic pressure) enhances superior and inferior vena cava (IVC) blood flows secondary to decreases in right atrial pressure (Pra) induced by a fall in the intrathoracic pressure.[1] However, during inspiration, descent of the diaphragm also causes changes in intra-abdominal pressure,[2] which may affect venous return in complex ways. The abdominal vascular compartment has a large capacitance and is directly upstream to the intrathoracic compartment. IVC venous return accounts for two-thirds of the systemic venous return and insight into factors influencing changes in IVC venous return is crucial.

Previous work documented conflicting results of the effect of increasing Pab on venous return. Many studies found that IVC venous return increased with rising Pab.[3–5] However, other investigators reported a decrease in venous return that was dependent on the magnitude of stress and conditions of the circulatory system.[6,7]

In 1964, West and colleagues[8] proposed the pulmonary vascular zone theory to explain the relationships between pulmonary blood flow, vascular pressures, and alveolar pressures. To reconcile differences in observations of the influence of Pab on venous return Takata and colleagues[9] (analogous to West zones) put forth the concept of presence of similar vascular zones in the abdomen. In this elegant model, they hypothesized that a vascular waterfall[10] would develop within the IVC at the level of the diaphragm and that the occurrence of such a waterfall was dependent on pressure within the abdomen (Pab), pressure within the abdominal IVC (Pivc), and the critical transmural closing pressure of the IVC at the waterfall (Pc). In earlier work Lloyd[4] had demonstrated that flow in the abdominal IVC was in the forward direction unless Pivc was 5 cm $H_2O$ or more below Pab and concluded that rather than behaving as a pure Starling resistor, the IVC had a tethering open capacity of Pc. Takata's model is illustrated in **Fig. 1**, wherein there is an upstream extra-abdominal venous compartment (Vu) and a downstream abdominal compartment (Vb), which is surrounded by Pab. Both empty into the thoracic IVC. Using this model, Takata and colleagues described two resting abdominal zone conditions: zone 2 and zone 3. In zone 3, IVC pressure at the level of diaphragm (Pivc) exceeds the sum of Pab and critical closing Pc. In this case, the effective back pressure to IVC flow is Pivc. In zone 2 conditions the sum of Pc and Pab is greater than Pivc and the effective backpressure to IVC flow is Pab + Pc. Changing Pab depending on initial resting state of the abdomen results in one of three scenarios: (1) zone 3 conditions are maintained with increase of Pab, (2) zone 2 conditions are maintained with increase of Pab, and (3) the abdomen transitions to zone 2 state from zone 3 after application of an increase in Pab. In the first scenario (zone 3 to zone 3), backpressure to IVC flow would not change but blood would be discharged from the abdominal compartment because of increased Pab, whereas blood volume in the extra-abdominal compartment would remain the same (extra-abdominal compartment, which is not surrounded by Pab, effectively sees Pivc as the back pressure), leading to a decrease in the total IVC volume. In the second

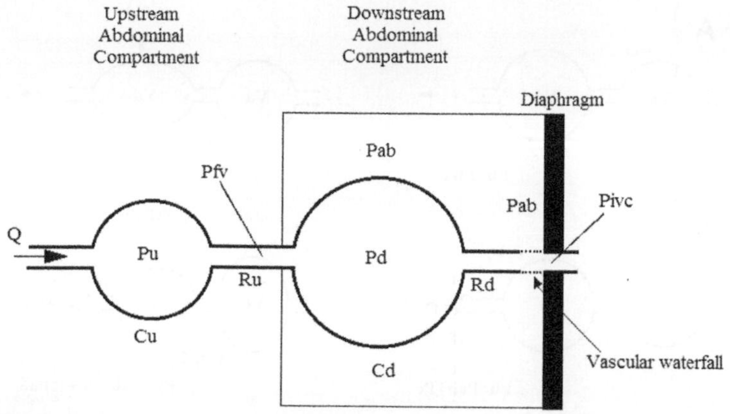


**Fig. 1.** Model of IVC. Cd, compliance in downstream compartment; Cu, compliance in upstream compartment; Pd, pressure in downstream compartment, Pfv, pressure in the femoral vein; Pu, pressure in upstream compartment; Rd - Resistance in downstream compartment; Ru- Resistance in upstream compartment. (*Adapted from* Takata M, Wise RA, Robotham JL. Effects of abdominal pressure on venous return: abdominal vascular zone conditions. J Appl Physiol (1985) 1990;69(6):1961–72.)

scenario (zone 2 to zone 2), increased Pab would increase backpressure for IVC flow, which would be offset by an equal increase in the pressure surrounding the abdominal compartment; however, backpressure for the extra-abdominal compartment would increase. Therefore there would be no change of volume in the abdominal compartment; however, blood would be trapped in the extra-abdominal compartment increasing the total blood volume within the IVC. In the last scenario (zone 3 to zone 2), a waterfall develops when the sum of Pab and Pc exceeds Pivc. Before reaching this waterfall blood is discharged from the abdominal compartment. Once the waterfall is reached, blood is trapped in the extra-abdominal compartment. The effect on the volume within the IVC is variable (increase, decrease, or no net change) depending on the initial conditions. These theoretic conditions are represented in **Fig. 2**.

To confirm their hypothetical model, Takata and colleagues performed a series of innovative experiments on 12 open-chested dogs with their IVC circulation bypassed by means of a cannula inserted into the IVC, 2 cm above the diaphragm. Pressure in the IVC was controlled with a Starling resistor and the authors tested their aforementioned theoretic model by varying Pivc, baseline Pab, and transiently increasing Pab via bilateral phrenic nerve stimulation. **Fig. 3** schematically represents their results. In **Fig. 3**A, Pivc is much larger than Pab at baseline and zone 3 conditions prevail; transiently increasing Pab with phrenic nerve stimulation increases IVC flow as predicted by their theoretic model. **Fig. 3**E representative of zone 2 conditions shows a fall in IVC flow with a transient increase in Pab and **Fig. 3**B–D reflect progressive conditions in which the zone 3 conditions change to zone 2 conditions and IVC flow increases to varying degrees and then falls, depending on the time point of transition from zone 3 to 2. The authors then confirmed their theory of the existence of a vascular waterfall at the thoracic inlet of the IVC by altering Pivc at different levels of Pab and measuring pressure in the femoral vein (Pfv), which is outside the abdominal cavity (**Fig. 4**). As demonstrated in **Fig. 4** at various levels of Pab (progressively decreasing from **Fig. 4**A–E), changing Pivc did not change Pfv (no reflection of pressure downstream of the waterfall to upstream components or zone 2) until a critical inflection point beyond which changes in Pivc mirrored changes in Pfv (reflection of pressure

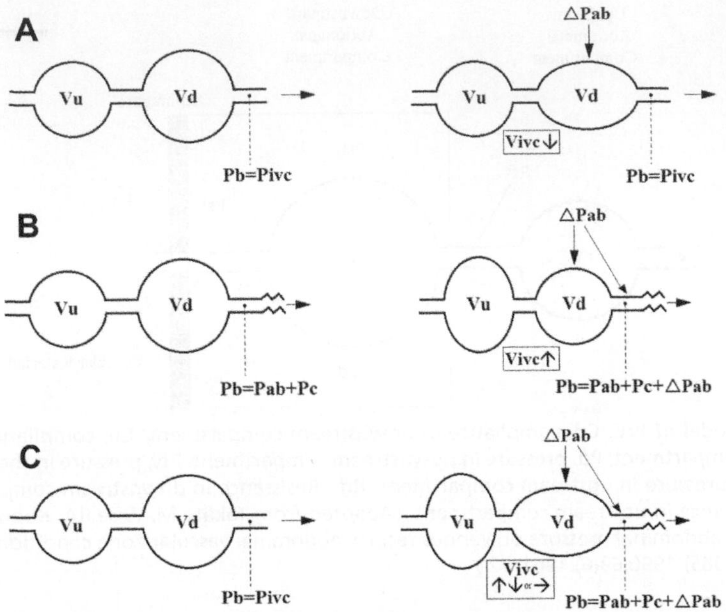


**Fig. 2.** Changes in blood volume in IVC circulation with increasing abdominal pressure. (*A*) Pure zone 3 abdomen. (*B*) Pure zone 2 abdomen. (*C*) Transition from zone 3 to zone 2 abdomen. Pb, back pressure to IVC flow at the thorax; Vd, blood volume in the downstream abdominal compartment; Vivc, volume within the IVC circulation; Vu, blood volume in the upstream extra-abdominal compartment. (*Adapted from* Takata M, Wise RA, Robotham JL. Effects of abdominal pressure on venous return: abdominal vascular zone conditions. J Appl Physiol (1985) 1990;69(6):1961–72.)

downstream of the waterfall to upstream components or zone 3) and for each Pab, the portion of the curve beyond the inflection point was virtually superimposable. These results demonstrated that a vascular waterfall does indeed exist and the pressure at which this waterfall occurs depends on the relative values of Pab and Pivc.

In a subsequent set of elegant experiments, Takata and Robotham[11] isolated changes in Pab from changes in intrathoracic pressure using open-chested dogs rendered apneic. First they demonstrated that increases in Pab induced by phrenic

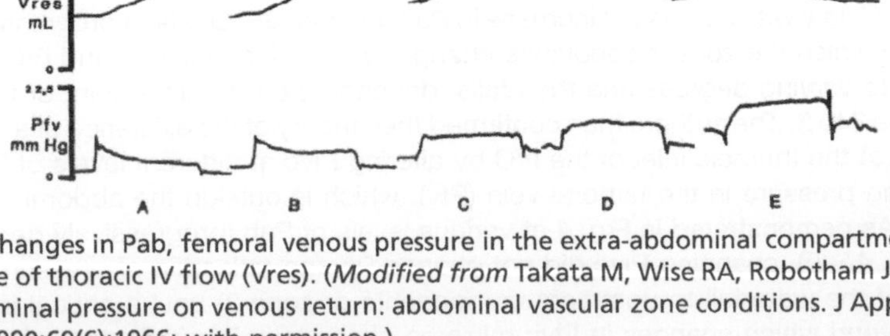

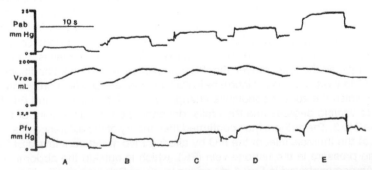


**Fig. 3.** Changes in Pab, femoral venous pressure in the extra-abdominal compartment (Pfv), and state of thoracic IV flow (Vres). (*Modified from* Takata M, Wise RA, Robotham JL. Effects of abdominal pressure on venous return: abdominal vascular zone conditions. J Appl Physiol (1985) 1990;69(6):1966; with permission.)

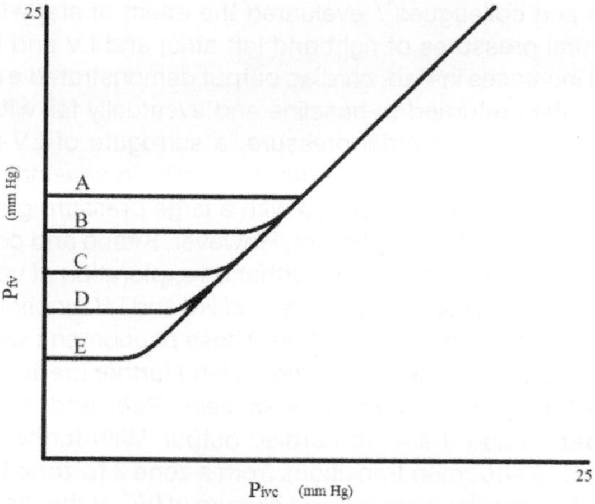


**Fig. 4.** Femoral vein pressure versus IVC pressure at different levels of Pab. (*Adapted from* Takata M, Wise RA, Robotham JL. Effects of abdominal pressure on venous return: abdominal vascular zone conditions. J Appl Physiol (1985) 1990;69(6):1961–72.)

nerve stimulation causing diaphragmatic descent increased thoracic IVC flow in hypervolemic animals and the source of the increased flow was mainly the splanchnic venous vasculature. Further in hypervolemic animals, Pra was always higher than Pab even when Pab was transiently increased during phrenic nerve stimulation. Conversely in hypovolemic animals, increases in Pab first transiently increased and then caused a sustained decrease in IVC flow. In these hypovolemic animals, Pab exceeded Pra during phrenic nerve stimulation indicating development of zone 2 conditions; decreased IVC flow was mostly through a reduction in nonsplanchnic IVC flow. In another set of experiments Fessler and colleagues[12] demonstrated pressure drops at a discreet point in the thoracic IVC on application of PEEP. This pressure drop could be overcome by volume loading to raise intravascular pressure and then reproduced by raising PEEP to increase extravascular pressure. These results suggest that changes in venous return observed with PEEP may be explained by changes in Pab and development of a vascular waterfall at the IVC near the thoracic inlet. Regardless of the cause, the effect on venous return induced by PEEP or positive pressure ventilation can be overcome with adequate blood volume expansion.

## RELATIONSHIP BETWEEN VENTRICULAR FUNCTION AND ABDOMINAL PRESSURE

Previous studies demonstrated that increasing Pab depressed cardiac output; however, the mechanism of depression is still a matter of intense debate.[13–16] Kashtan and colleagues[15] found that increasing Pab to 40 mm Hg increased systemic vascular resistance (SVR), depressed the left ventricle (LV) function curve, and impaired right ventricle (RV) performance. They surmised that the depression in cardiac output was secondary to increased SVR. Bloomfield and colleagues[13] in a swine model studied the effects of increasing Pab to 25 mm Hg and included a group of animals that underwent sternotomy and pleuropericardotomy to negate increases in pleural pressure caused by increasing Pab. In their model cardiac output fell regardless of whether or not the animals were close chested. However, there were some studies that demonstrated a rise in cardiac output on increasing Pab. To reconcile these differences, Kitano and colleagues[17] evaluated the effect of stepwise increments of Pab on the transmural pressures of right and left atria, and LV and RV function.

With incremental increases in Pab, cardiac output demonstrated a biphasic change. It increased initially, then returned to baseline and eventually fell with progressive increases in Pab. Transmural left atrial pressure, a surrogate of LV preload, demonstrated a response similar to cardiac output, initially increasing and then falling. When cardiac output fell, it was associated with a large pressure gradient that developed in the IVC at the level of the diaphragm. However, Kitano and colleagues[17] found that the transmural Pra consistently rose. Further on exploration of ventricular function curves, they found that increasing Pab depressed RV and LV function curves, with the RV function more depressed than LV function. These phenomena were attributable to a rise in RV and LV afterload. These experiments lend further credence to the abdominal vascular zone theory. Initially the Pra exceeds Pab, and an increase in Pab increases venous return and therefore cardiac output. With further increase in Pab, Pra falls below Pab, the abdomen transitions from a zone 3 to zone 2 conditions leading to the creation of a vascular waterfall and closure of IVC at the diaphragm and large pressure difference between the IVC and Pra. This leads to a reduction in the venous return (**Fig. 5**). These data support the notion that when Pab increases sufficiently, depression of cardiac output is secondary to a decrement in venous return and an increment in the afterload of the RV and LV. These afterload increments are likely secondary to compression of the small pulmonary and systemic arterial vasculature.

## CLINICAL APPLICATIONS

### *Prone Positioning*

The PROSEVA trial[18] demonstrated that early applications of prone positioning (PP) was associated with a significant reduction in mortality in patients with severe acute respiratory distress syndrome (ARDS). This effect is likely from improvement in alveolar recruitment and reduction in regional overdistention of the lung.[19] PP also promotes a more homogenous distribution of transpulmonary pressure along the

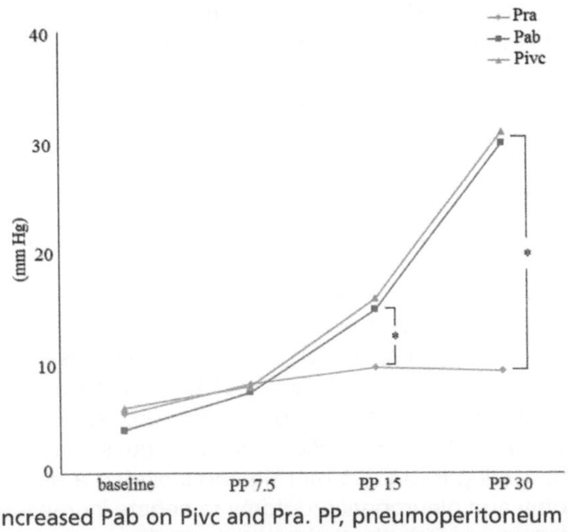


**Fig. 5.** Effects of increased Pab on Pivc and Pra. PP, pneumoperitoneum created to increase abdominal pressure progressively from baseline to 30 mm Hg. (*Adapted from* Kitano Y, Takata M, Sasaki N, et al. Influence of increased abdominal pressure on steady-state cardiac performance. J Appl Physiol (1985) 1999;86(5):1651–6.)

ventral to dorsal axis.[20] However, one important aspect that is often overlooked is the influence of PP on Pab and consequent impact on systemic hemodynamics. Furthermore, the effect of ARDS on thoracoabdominal compliance and Pab depends on whether the ARDS is pulmonary or extrapulmonary.[21–23] Extrapulmonary causes of ARDS are usually associated with higher intra-abdominal pressure and greater amounts of collapsed and recruitable lung.[22,24]

Most human studies report a rise in Pab when position is switched from supine to prone.[25–28] However, outcome data are limited. Importantly none of the studies included patients with marked elevations of Pab. Furthermore, an integrated view of the physiologic effects of increased Pab has rarely been reported.

In a recent study, Jozwiak and colleagues[29] studied the hemodynamic effects of PP in patients with ARDS. They included 18 patients with ARDS with a mean baseline P/F ratio of 134. Passive leg raise test was done to ascertain preload reserve (defined as >10% increase in cardiac index on passive leg raise). These investigators found that Pab increased in all patients after PP. Moreover, PP increased the cardiac index by more than 15% in patients with preload reserve, whereas in patients who did not have preload reserve the cardiac index did not change significantly. These findings are consistent with the vascular zone theory proposed by Takata and colleagues. All patients had high Pra and Pab was consistently lower than Pra. Therefore, zone 3 conditions were prevalent (Pra > Pab + Pc), and an increase in the Pab on PP increased the venous return. PP did not increase the Pab enough to switch them to zone 2 conditions (**Table 1**).

Importantly none of their patients had very high Pab at baseline. Although unknown, it is reasonable to hypothesize that if the Pra < Pab + Pc (zone 2 conditions), such as in cases with elevated intra-abdominal pressure or intra-abdominal hypertension, PP would lead to creation of a waterfall, collapsing the IVC and reducing venous return to the RA.

In their study, Jozwiak and colleagues[29] found that pulmonary vascular resistance significantly decreased in all patients, whereas the LV afterload (mean arterial pressure and product of LV end-systolic area and systolic arterial pressure) significantly increased. It is likely that in their patients without significant intra-abdominal hypertension, the beneficial effects of PP on pulmonary vascular resistance were far greater in magnitude than the adverse effects of increased Pab.

Although never evaluated, it is probably reasonable to surmise that in patients who do have more than mild elevations of Pab (morbidly obese patients, patients with intra-abdominal hypertension, or patients with low abdominal compliance) that PP may adversely affect hemodynamics by impairing venous return and causing RV

**Table 1**
**Effect of Prone Positioning on Pra, Pab, and Cardiac index in patients with and without preload reserve**

| | No Preload Reserve, Supine | No Preload Reserve, Prone | Preload Reserve, Supine | Preload Reserve, Prone |
|---|---|---|---|---|
| Pra | 10 | 16 | 15 | 17 |
| Pab | 14 | 17 | 16 | 18 |
| Cardiac index | 3.2 | 3.3 | 3.0 | 3.6 |

*Adapted from* Jozwiak M, Teboul JL, Anguel N, et al. Beneficial hemodynamic effects of prone positioning in patients with acute respiratory distress syndrome. Am J Respir Crit Care Med 2013;188(12):1428–33.

dysfunction. In such circumstances blood volume expansion can potentially lead to further worsening of RV function. We therefore suggest that intra-abdominal pressure be monitored before and during PP. In cases where intra-abdominal pressure is increased and PP is required, it may be prudent to use gravitational abdominal unloading techniques, such as thoracopelvic supports to suspend the abdomen to fully realize the benefits of PP.[30]

### *Ascites*

Large-volume paracentesis are frequently avoided in patients with cirrhosis with ascites secondary to the risk of precipitating postparacentesis circulatory dysfunction.[31,32] The mechanisms of postparacentesis circulatory dysfunction, however, are not well elucidated. Most studies report that in cirrhosis with tense ascites large-volume paracentesis progressively lowers Pab and increases cardiac index or stroke volume.[31,33–35] Pozzi and colleagues[35] performed a careful immediate and longer term hemodynamic study in 12 patients in cirrhosis and tense ascites. On rapid removal of ascites (approximately 10 L over 1 hour), they found that both intra-abdominal and intrathoracic pressure declined. The Pra also declined significantly but the transmural Pra did not change, suggesting a removal of a mechanical obstruction to venous return. Furthermore, in their study, SVR declined significantly with a concomitant rise in stroke volume index. Despite these beneficial effects, mean arterial pressure fell significantly because the rise in cardiac index was inadequate to counterbalance the fall in SVR. Parallel to this study, Cabrera and colleagues[36] studied 11 patients with tense ascites receiving large-volume paracentesis. They used a pneumatic girdle to compress the abdomen to avoid decreases in Pab during the paracentesis. They observed no hemodynamic changes when Pab was held constant but SVR declined once the pneumatic girdle was released. They concluded that abrupt decreases in Pab were responsible for the hemodynamic changes observed with large-volume paracentesis. Similarly, Coll and colleagues[37] found that a higher baseline intra-abdominal pressure, shorter duration of paracentesis, and higher flow rate of ascites extraction were associated with significant decline in SVR.

Kravetz and colleagues[38] reported a significant fall in variceal size, variceal diameter, and wall tension after large-volume paracentesis. Luca and colleagues[39] demonstrated that increasing Pab in patients with cirrhosis with portal hypertension leads to a fall in cardiac output, rise in SVR, and rise in mean arterial pressure. Furthermore, hepatic venous pressure and portal pressure rose with increases in Pab. Concomitantly hepatic blood flow decreased, accompanied by an increase in the azygous blood flow (surrogate for gastroesophageal collateral blood flow).

These data suggest that cardiac output rises with large-volume paracentesis but is not adequate to counteract the systemic vasodilation that simultaneously occurs. The consequence is decreased mean arterial pressure. The mechanism of the fall in SVR may be mechanical from relief of increased Pab or secondary to neurohormonal changes. The exact mechanism is still a matter of debate. Finally, increased Pab with ascites may result in increased portocollateral flow and increase in variceal size. Therefore, large-volume paracentesis may have many beneficial effects if sudden decreases in Pab are avoided.[40] Consideration should be given to volume expansion using albumin[41] or alternatively using vasoconstrictor agents[42,43] concomitantly with large-volume paracentesis.

### *Laparoscopic Surgery*

Intra-abdominal insufflation during laparoscopic surgery raises the Pab to approximately 15 mm Hg.[44,45] Although not exceedingly elevated, this degree of Pab elevation may have deleterious clinical consequences especially in patients with overt/occult cardiac dysfunction.

Gebhardt and colleagues[45] studied 15 patients with pre-existing cardiac dysfunction who underwent $CO_2$ insufflation to 14 mm Hg. As in previous studies they found that as Pab increased Pra similarly increased. However, this was accompanied by greater increases in esophageal pressure (surrogate of pleural pressure) and the calculated transmural pressure actually declined. Similar to previous studies, stroke volume fell and SVR increased. The observed changes in right atrial and transmural Pra were completely reversible on abdominal decompression. The increases in Pra were a direct consequence of the transmission on increased Pab to the thoracic cavity. It is plausible that the fall in transmural Pra was secondary to creation of zone 2 conditions in the abdomen and decrements in venous return. Regardless, these findings suggest that use of right atrial or pulmonary capillary wedge pressures with increases in Pab is potentially misleading and caution should be exercised in their interpretation. Moreover, even modest elevations of Pab have the potential to deleteriously affect circulatory physiology and intensivists should be aware of these complex interactions. These deleterious effects are likely to be magnified in patients who have compromised RV or LV function at baseline, where further alterations in preload and afterload may cause frank RV or LV failure in a marginal ventricle without reserve.

### *Weaning from Mechanical Ventilation*

Application of positive pressure ventilation, especially with PEEP, results in an increase in the Pab.[46] This is likely secondary to the transmission of increased intrathoracic pressure to the abdomen and the caudal displacement of the diaphragm. Conversely, elevated Pab is transmitted to the thorax and may negatively affect cardiac and respiratory performance. Both aspects may be important when switching from positive pressure breathing to spontaneous breathing, as during a weaning trial. During mechanical ventilation with the diaphragm relaxed, the increase in intrathoracic pressure is likely transmitted to the abdomen with little or no increase in transdiaphragmatic pressure. However, during spontaneous respiration, intrathoracic pressure falls while Pab increases causing an increase in the transdiaphragmatic pressure. Hence under zone 3 conditions of the abdomen, during positive pressure ventilation the gradient for venous return to the thorax (Pivc – Pra) does not change. However, during spontaneous respiration under zone 3 conditions, the gradient for venous return increases. This is probably the elegant physiology at work in a landmark paper from Lemaire and colleagues,[47] which first described weaning-induced cardiac dysfunction. In this study, the authors detailed hemodynamics of 15 patients with severe chronic obstructive pulmonary disease undergoing a weaning trial. They found that unsuccessful weaning trials were all associated with marked increases in transmural pulmonary artery occlusion pressure (PAOP) with unchanged RV and LV systolic function. Once these patients shed approximately 5 kg in weight by diuresis, weaning was successful. Interestingly, unsuccessful weaning was also accompanied by large rises in transmural Pra. This rise in transmural Pra was much greater than the fall in pleural pressure that occurred during spontaneously ventilation. Lemaire and colleagues[47] posited that an increase in preload and LV afterload that accompanied the switch from positive to negative pressure breathing was the mechanism of their observations. However, the magnitude of the rise in transmural Pra beyond the fall in pleural pressure is counterintuitive because a fall in Pra is the driving force for increased venous return in the first place. These findings may be reconciled by considering Pab and transdiaphragmatic pressure as articulated in a brilliant editorial by Permutt.[48] He surmised that during positive pressure ventilation, transdiaphragmatic pressure would not change, but on switching to spontaneous respiration Pra would fall. Simultaneously, Pab would rise around an engorged splanchnic vasculature resulting in marked increases in preload. Diuresis effectively reduced blood volume in the splanchnic vasculature resulting in decreased abdominal blood flow into the thoracic cavity, resulting in successful weaning. Although Pab was not measured in the study conducted by Lemaire and colleagues,[47] Pemutt's remarkable insights were borne out when Takata and colleagues[49] later demonstrated that the pathogenesis of the Kussmaul sign (paradoxic inspiratory increase in Pra seen in pericardial disease) was secondary to a much larger increase in Pab relative to fall in intrathoracic pressure under conditions of hypervolemia, causing increased venous return. In another recent study, Lamia and colleagues[50] investigated the value of echocardiography in detecting elevations of PAOP in patients who failed spontaneous breathing trials. Similar to Lemaire and colleagues[47] they observed that in patients whose PAOP rose to 18 mm Hg and above during the weaning trial, Pra also rose markedly. In his accompanying editorial, Fessler[51] argued that because stroke volume index was unchanged and pulmonary artery pressure rose as well, it was unlikely that increased Pab and increases in venous return could explain these findings. He proposed a rise in pleural pressure because of dynamic hyperinflation or recruitment of expiratory muscles as a unifying mechanism of the observed phenomena. However, on careful observation of the data, in the cohort that experienced a rise in PAOP, in addition to rise in Pra, pulmonary artery pressure and systemic mean arterial pressure rose as well. Moreover, despite the unchanged stroke volume index, ejection fraction actually fell (although this did not reach statistical significance). The unchanged stroke volume with a fall in ejection fraction is highly suggestive of an increase in preload with the heart functioning at the flat portion of the Frank-Starling curve. Increase in pulmonary artery and a systemic blood pressure suggests increases in afterload, all consequences of increasing Pab.

## SUMMARY

There are considerable effects of increased Pab on circulatory and respiratory physiology even in the absence of intra-abdominal hypertension. These effects are in play in a variety of common clinical conditions including ascites, transitioning from positive pressure to spontaneous breathing, transmission of Pab to the intrathoracic compartment and cardiac chambers, measurement of static pressures within cardiac chambers, and positioning of patients with ARDS. Intensivists should have a fundamental understanding of these effects and take them into account when making hemodynamic decisions in critically ill patients.

## REFERENCES


1. Guyton AC. Determination of cardiac output by equating venous return curves with cardiac response curves. Physiol Rev 1955;35(1):123–9.
2. Decramer M, De Troyer A, Kelly S, et al. Regional differences in abdominal pressure swings in dogs. J Appl Physiol Respir Environ Exerc Physiol 1984; 57(6):1682–7.
3. Eckstein RW, Wiggers CJ, Graham GR. Phasic changes in inferior cava flow of intravascular origin. Am J Physiol 1947;148(3):740–4.
4. Lloyd TC Jr. Effect of inspiration on inferior vena caval blood flow in dogs. J Appl Physiol Respir Environ Exerc Physiol 1983;55(6):1701–8.
5. Moreno AH, Burchell AR, Van der Woude R, et al. Respiratory regulation of splanchnic and systemic venous return. Am J Physiol 1967;213(2):455–65.

6. Smith HJ, Grøttum P, Simonsen S. Ultrasonic assessment of abdominal venous return. I. Effect of cardiac action and respiration on mean velocity pattern, cross-sectional area and flow in the inferior vena cava and portal vein. Acta Radiol Diagn (Stockh) 1985;26(5):581–8.
7. Wexler L, Bergel DH, Gabe IT, et al. Velocity of blood flow in normal human venae cavae. Circ Res 1968;23(3):349–59.
8. West JB, Dollery CT, Naimark A. Distribution of blood flow in isolated lung; relation to vascular and alveolar pressure. J Appl Physiol 1964;19:713–24.
9. Takata M, Wise RA, Robotham JL. Effects of abdominal pressure on venous return: abdominal vascular zone conditions. J Appl Physiol (1985) 1990;69(6):1961–72.
10. Permutt S, Riley RL. Hemodynamics of collapsible vessels with tone: the vascular waterfall. J Appl Physiol 1963;18:924–32.
11. Takata M, Robotham JL. Effects of inspiratory diaphragmatic descent on inferior vena caval venous return. J Appl Physiol (1985) 1992;72(2):597–607.
12. Fessler HE, Brower RG, Shapiro EP, et al. Effects of positive end-expiratory pressure and body position on pressure in the thoracic great veins. Am Rev Respir Dis 1993;148(6 Pt 1):1657–64.
13. Bloomfield GL, Ridings PC, Blocher CR, et al. A proposed relationship between increased intra-abdominal, intrathoracic, and intracranial pressure. Crit Care Med 1997;25(3):496–503.
14. Ridings PC, Bloomfield GL, Blocher CR, et al. Cardiopulmonary effects of raised intra-abdominal pressure before and after intravascular volume expansion. J Trauma 1995;39(6):1071–5.
15. Kashtan J, Green JF, Parsons EQ, et al. Hemodynamic effect of increased abdominal pressure. J Surg Res 1981;30(3):249–55.
16. Robotham JL, Wise RA, Bromberger-Barnea B. Effects of changes in abdominal pressure on left ventricular performance and regional blood flow. Crit Care Med 1985;13(10):803–9.
17. Kitano Y, Takata M, Sasaki N, et al. Influence of increased abdominal pressure on steady-state cardiac performance. J Appl Physiol (1985) 1999;86(5):1651–6.
18. Guérin C, Reignier J, Richard JC, et al, PROSEVA Study Group. Prone positioning in severe acute respiratory distress syndrome. N Engl J Med 2013;368(23):2159–68.
19. Galiatsou E, Kostanti E, Svarna E, et al. Prone position augments recruitment and prevents alveolar overinflation in acute lung injury. Am J Respir Crit Care Med 2006;174(2):187–97.
20. Mutoh T, Guest RJ, Lamm WJ, et al. Prone position alters the effect of volume overload on regional pleural pressures and improves hypoxemia in pigs in vivo. Am Rev Respir Dis 1992;146(2):300–6.
21. Ranieri VM, Brienza N, Santostasi S, et al. Impairment of lung and chest wall mechanics in patients with acute respiratory distress syndrome: role of abdominal distension. Am J Respir Crit Care Med 1997;156(4 Pt 1):1082–91.
22. Gattinoni L, Pelosi P, Suter PM, et al. Acute respiratory distress syndrome caused by pulmonary and extrapulmonary disease. Different syndromes? Am J Respir Crit Care Med 1998;158(1):3–11.
23. Lim CM, Kim EK, Lee JS, et al. Comparison of the response to the prone position between pulmonary and extrapulmonary acute respiratory distress syndrome. Intensive Care Med 2001;27(3):477–85.
24. Riva DR, Oliveira MB, Rzezinski AF, et al. Recruitment maneuver in pulmonary and extrapulmonary experimental acute lung injury. Crit Care Med 2008;36(6):1900–8.

25. Pelosi P, Tubiolo D, Mascheroni D, et al. Effects of the prone position on respiratory mechanics and gas exchange during acute lung injury. Am J Respir Crit Care Med 1998;157(2):387–93.
26. Hering R, Wrigge H, Vorwerk R, et al. The effects of prone positioning on intraabdominal pressure and cardiovascular and renal function in patients with acute lung injury. Anesth Analg 2001;92(5):1226–31.
27. Hering R, Vorwerk R, Wrigge H, et al. Prone positioning, systemic hemodynamics, hepatic indocyanine green kinetics, and gastric intramucosal energy balance in patients with acute lung injury. Intensive Care Med 2002;28(1):53–8.
28. Michelet P, Roch A, Gainnier M, et al. Influence of support on intra-abdominal pressure, hepatic kinetics of indocyanine green and extravascular lung water during prone positioning in patients with ARDS: a randomized crossover study. Crit Care 2005;9(3):R251–7.
29. Jozwiak M, Teboul JL, Anguel N, et al. Beneficial hemodynamic effects of prone positioning in patients with acute respiratory distress syndrome. Am J Respir Crit Care Med 2013;188(12):1428–33.
30. Chiumello D, Cressoni M, Racagni M, et al. Effects of thoraco-pelvic supports during prone position in patients with acute lung injury/acute respiratory distress syndrome: a physiological study. Crit Care 2006;10(3):R87.
31. Knauer CM, Lowe HM. Hemodynamics in the cirrhotic patient during paracentesis. N Engl J Med 1967;276(9):491–6.
32. Kellerman PS, Linas SL. Large-volume paracentesis in treatment of ascites. Ann Intern Med 1990;112(12):889–91.
33. Savino JA, Cerabona T, Agarwal N, et al. Manipulation of ascitic fluid pressure in cirrhotics to optimize hemodynamic and renal function. Ann Surg 1988;208(4):504–11.
34. Guazzi M, Polese A, Magrini F, et al. Negative influences of ascites on the cardiac function of cirrhotic patients. Am J Med 1975;59(2):165–70.
35. Pozzi M, Osculati G, Boari G, et al. Time course of circulatory and humoral effects of rapid total paracentesis in cirrhotic patients with tense, refractory ascites. Gastroenterology 1994;106(3):709–19.
36. Cabrera J, Falcón L, Gorriz E, et al. Abdominal decompression plays a major role in early postparacentesis haemodynamic changes in cirrhotic patients with tense ascites. Gut 2001;48(3):384–9.
37. Coll S, Vila MC, Molina L, et al. Mechanisms of early decrease in systemic vascular resistance after total paracentesis: influence of flow rate of ascites extraction. Eur J Gastroenterol Hepatol 2004;16(3):347–53.
38. Kravetz D, Romero G, Argonz J, et al. Total volume paracentesis decreases variceal pressure, size, and variceal wall tension in cirrhotic patients. Hepatology 1997;25(1):59–62.
39. Luca A, Cirera I, García-Pagán JC, et al. Hemodynamic effects of acute changes in intra-abdominal pressure in patients with cirrhosis. Gastroenterology 1993; 104(1):222–7.
40. Sen Sarma M, Yachha SK, Bhatia V, et al. Safety, complications and outcome of large volume paracentesis with or without albumin therapy in children with severe ascites due to liver disease. J Hepatol 2015;63(5):1126–32.
41. Ginès P, Titó L, Arroyo V, et al. Randomized comparative study of therapeutic paracentesis with and without intravenous albumin in cirrhosis. Gastroenterology 1988;94(6):1493–502.
42. Moreau R, Asselah T, Condat B, et al. Comparison of the effect of terlipressin and albumin on arterial blood volume in patients with cirrhosis and tense ascites treated by paracentesis: a randomised pilot study. Gut 2002;50(1):90–4.

43. Saló J, Ginès A, Ginès P, et al. Effect of therapeutic paracentesis on plasma volume and transvascular escape rate of albumin in patients with cirrhosis. J Hepatol 1997;27(4):645–53.
44. Myre K, Buanes T, Smith G, et al. Simultaneous hemodynamic and echocardiographic changes during abdominal gas insufflation. Surg Laparosc Endosc 1997;7(5):415–9.
45. Gebhardt H, Bautz A, Ross M, et al. Pathophysiological and clinical aspects of the CO2 pneumoperitoneum (CO2-PP). Surg Endosc 1997;11(8):864–7.
46. Soler Morejón Cde D, Tamargo Barbeito TO. Effect of mechanical ventilation on intra-abdominal pressure in critically ill patients without other risk factors for abdominal hypertension: an observational multicenter epidemiological study. Ann Intensive Care 2012;2(Suppl 1):S22.
47. Lemaire F, Teboul JL, Cinotti L, et al. Acute left ventricular dysfunction during unsuccessful weaning from mechanical ventilation. Anesthesiology 1988;69(2): 171–9.
48. Permutt S. Circulatory effects of weaning from mechanical ventilation: the importance of transdiaphragmatic pressure. Anesthesiology 1988;69(2):157–60.
49. Takata M, Beloucif S, Shimada M, et al. Superior and inferior vena caval flows during respiration: pathogenesis of Kussmaul's sign. Am J Physiol 1992; 262(3 Pt 2):H763–70.
50. Lamia B, Maizel J, Ochagavia A, et al. Echocardiographic diagnosis of pulmonary artery occlusion pressure elevation during weaning from mechanical ventilation. Crit Care Med 2009;37(5):1696–701.
51. Fessler HE. The cycles of heart, lungs, and science. Crit Care Med 2009;37(5): 1816–7.

# Severe Acute Pancreatitis and Necrotizing Pancreatitis

Rahul Maheshwari, MD[a,*], Ram M. Subramanian, MD[b]

**KEYWORDS**

- Acute pancreatitis • Necrotizing pancreatitis • Mortality • Morbidity

**KEY POINTS**

- Acute pancreatitis varies widely in its clinical presentation, from clinically neglible to precipitiously fatal despite any intervention.
- Necrotizing pancreatitis is a manifestation of severe acute pancreatitis and is associated with significant morbidity and mortality.
- Having established the diagnosis of pancreatic necrosis, goals of appropriately aggressive resuscitation should be established and adhered to in a multidisciplinary approach involving medical and surgical intensive care.
- In all cases of necrotizing pancreatitis, a multidisciplinary approach is needed, using endoscopic techniques and/or percutaneous drainage.
- Open surgery should be reserved for failure of less invasive techniques.

## INTRODUCTION

Acute pancreatitis results in nearly 250,000 annual admissions at a cost of approximately \$2.2 billion.[1,2] In most cases, acute pancreatitis represents a mild, self-limited disease, but in 15% to 25%, severe acute pancreatitis (SAP) develops, manifested with pancreatic parenchymal and/or peripancreatic tissue necrosis.[3] Pancreatic necrosis accounts for substantial additional morbidity, with mortality remaining as high as 10% to 20% despite advances in critical care.[4,5]

### *Severe Acute Pancreatitis*

Acute pancreatitis is best defined clinically by a patient presenting with 2 of the following 3 criteria: (1) symptoms (eg, epigastric pain) consistent with pancreatitis;

Disclosures: None.

[a] Division of Digestive Diseases, Emory University School of Medicine, 615 Michael Street, Suite 201, Atlanta, GA 30302, USA; [b] Emory University School of Medicine, 1365 Clifton Road NE, B6100, Atlanta, GA 30322
* Corresponding author.
*E-mail address:* rahul.maheshwari@emory.edu

Crit Care Clin 32 (2016) 279–290
http://dx.doi.org/10.1016/j.ccc.2015.12.006 criticalcare.theclinics.com
0749-0704/16/\$ – see front matter 

(2) a serum amylase or lipase level greater than 3 times the laboratory's upper limit of normal; and (3) radiologic imaging consistent with pancreatitis, usually computed tomography (CT) or MRI. Once the diagnosis of acute pancreatitis is established, patients are classified based on disease severity. The Atlanta Criteria revision of 2012 (**Box 1**)[6] classifies severity as mild, moderately severe, or severe. Severe acute pancreatitis is defined by persistent single or multiorgan failure (lasting >48 hours). Local complications include peripancreatic fluid collections, pancreatic and peripancreatic necrosis (sterile or infected), pseudocyst, and wall-off necrosis (sterile or infected; **Figs. 1** and **2**).[6]

Other acceptable markers of severe pancreatitis include 3 or more of Ranson's II criteria for non-gallstone pancreatitis, and an Acute Physiology and Chronic Health Evaluation score greater than 8. It is important to use precise terms in describing the anatomic complications of acute pancreatitis. Although patients with interstitial pancreatitis have a normally perfused gland, manifesting on contrast-enhanced CT as normal, bright appears as an indication of flow throughout the gland; patients with necrotizing pancreatitis (NP) have greater than 30% of the gland that is not perfused, with low attenuation. Pancreatic necrosis is consistent with focal or diffuse nonviable pancreatic parenchyma and is usually accompanied by peripancreatic fat necrosis. Pancreatic necrosis can be sterile or infected. Peripancreatic necrosis describes necrotic fatty and tissue debris around the pancreas; it is more important to surgeons because this is typically not appreciated on imaging. NP (pancreatic necrosis) is defined, in the absence of laparotomy or autopsy, by the presence of greater than 30% of nonenhancement of the pancreas on a contrast-enhanced CT (or MRI with gadolinium). The determination that a patient has pancreatic necrosis has clinical implications because the morbidity and mortality of NP are higher than that associated with interstitial pancreatitis. Patients with NP may seem ill with single- or multiorgan failure or may seem well with no evidence of organ failure.

More recently, the 2012 revised Atlanta classification for acute pancreatitis addressed several lingering deficiencies and further developed consistent terminology for acute pancreatitis and its sequelae as highlighted in **Table 1**.[7] The term mild acute pancreatitis is now defined as pancreatitis without organ failure (defined in later discussion, such as renal or pulmonary failure), or complications (such as necrosis or

**Box 1**
**2012 Atlanta classification revision of acute pancreatitis**

*Definitions of grades and severity of acute pancreatitis*

Mild acute pancreatitis
  No organ failure
  No local or systemic complications

Moderately SAP
  Transient organ failure (<48 hours) and/or
  Local or systemic complications[a] without persistent organ failure

Severe acute pancreatitis
  Persistent organ failure (>48 hours)—single organ or multiorgan

[a] Local complications are peripancreatic fluid collections, pancreatic necrosis, and peripancreatic necrosis (sterile or infected), pseudocyst, and WON (sterile or infected).

*From* Banks PA, Bollen TL, Dervenis C, et al. Classification of acute pancreatitis—2012: revision of classification and definitions by international consensus. Gut 2013;62:102–11; with permission.

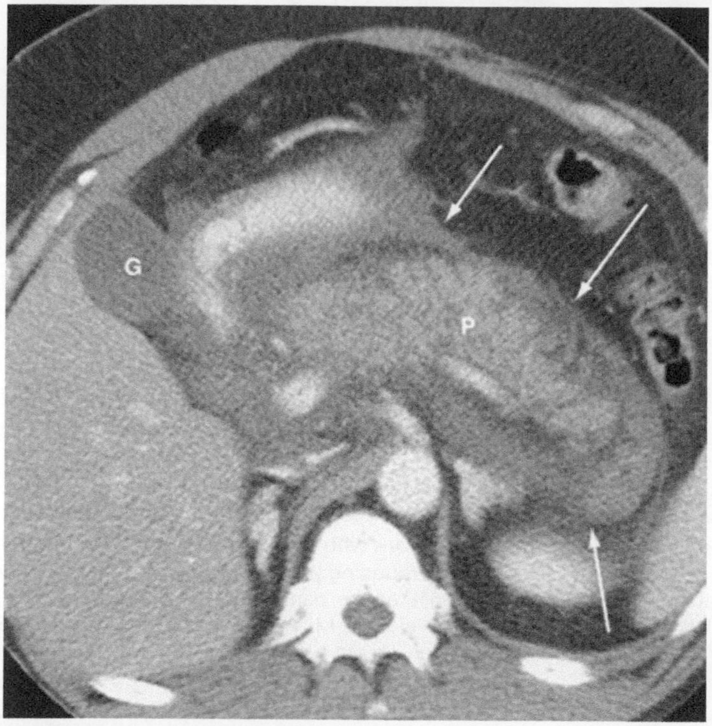


**Fig. 1.** CT showing acute interstitial pancreatitis with diffuse swelling of the pancreas (P) and peripancreatic inflammatory changes (*arrows*). The pancreas was well perfused without evidence of necrosis. G, gallbladder. (*From* Tenner S, Steinberg WM. Acute pancreatitis. In: Feldman M, Friedman LS, Brandt LJ, eds. Sleisenger and Fordtran's gastrointestinal and liver disease pathophysiology, diagnosis, management. 10th edition. Philadelphia: Elsevier; 2016; with permission.)

pseudocysts), as discussed later. Moderately severe acute pancreatitis is defined by organ failure lasting less than 48 hours, or by local complications. The term SAP is reserved for cases in which organ failure lasts greater than 48 hours. According to the current classification of acute pancreatitis, interstitial edematous pancreatitis (IEP) is defined by the lack of pancreatic or peripancreatic necrosis on imaging and is distinguished from NP, which is subdivided into 3 categories: parenchymal necrosis, peripancreatic necrosis, or combined necrosis, all 3 of which may be infected or sterile. The disease process is further separated into an early phase and a late phase, with definition of local complications based on characteristics of collections of fluid and necrosis. In the setting acute pancreatitis, typically IEP, a peripancreatic fluid collection occurring within the first 4 weeks is termed an acute peripancreatic fluid collection (APFC) and is characterized by the lack of both a well-defined wall and a pancreatic or peripancreatic necrosis on imaging. When an APFC persists beyond 4 weeks, a well-defined wall will develop, and the term pancreatic pseudocyst (PP) is applied. Similarly, in the setting of NP, a collection of not only fluid but also necrosis involving the pancreatic parenchyma or the peripancreatic tissues is termed an acute necrotic collection (ANC) when seen within the first 4 weeks of the disease. Like APFCs, ANCs lack a well-defined wall. When an ANC persists beyond 4 weeks and becomes encapsulated, the term walled-off necrosis (WON) is used. Concisely, an APFC contains no

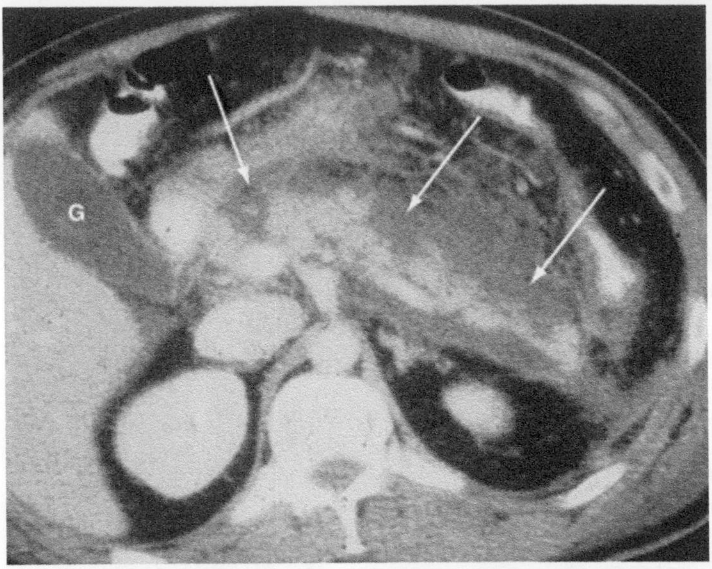


**Fig. 2.** CT showing acute pancreatic necrosis with focal areas of decreased perfusion in the pancreatic parenchyma (*arrows*) and surrounding peripancreatic inflammation. The necrosis was estimated to involve less than 30% of the pancreas. G, gallbladder. (*From* Tenner S, Steinberg WM. Acute pancreatitis. In: Feldman M, Friedman LS, Brandt LJ, eds. Sleisenger and Fordtran's gastrointestinal and liver disease pathophysiology, diagnosis, management. 10th edition. Philadelphia: Elsevier; 2016; with permission.)

**Table 1**
**Glossary of terminology**

| Term | Definition |
|---|---|
| Mild acute pancreatitis | Pancreatitis without evidence of organ failure or complications |
| Moderately severe acute pancreatitis | Pancreatitis with a local complication, such as APFC, PP, ANC, or WON (defined below) or with organ failure (defined below) lasting <48 h |
| SAP | Pancreatitis with a local complication, such as APFC, PP, ANC, or WON (defined below) or with organ failure (defined below) lasting more than 48 h |
| IEP | Pancreatitis that lacks pancreatic or peripancreatic necrosis on imaging |
| NP | Pancreatitis with parenchymal, peripancreatic, or combined necrosis, identified by contrast-enhanced imaging |
| APFC | Peripancreatic fluid collection that occurs within the first 4 wk of pancreatitis in the setting of IEP, without a well-defined wall |
| PP | APFC that has persisted more than 4 wk and now has evidence of well-defined wall |
| ANC | Collection of both fluid and necrotic solid material, in NP, within the first 4 wk, without a well-defined wall |
| WON | ANC that has persisted more than 4 wk and has developed a well-defined wall |
| Organ failure | A score of 2 or more for any organ system in the Marshall scoring system (see text) |

See text for further explanation.

*From* Sabo A, Goussous N, Sardana N, et al. Necrotizing pancreatitis: a review of multidisciplinary management. JOP 2015;16(2):126; with permission.

necrotic material, whereas ANC contains fluid and necrosis; when these 2 entities persist beyond 4 weeks, they become PP and WON, respectively. Erstwhile terms, such as pancreatic abscess, pancreatic sequestration, necroma, and organized pancreatic necrosis, have fallen out of favor, and their use should be discouraged to avoid confusion.[7]

## PATIENT EVALUATION OVERVIEW

### *Clinical Features*

#### *History*

Abdominal pain is present at the onset of most attacks of acute pancreatitis. Pain in pancreatitis usually involves the entire upper abdomen. However, it may be epigastric, in the right upper quadrant, or infrequently, confined to the left side. Onset of pain is rapid but not as abrupt as that of a perforated viscus. Usually, it is at maximal intensity in 10 to 20 minutes. Occasionally, pain gradually increases and takes several hours to reach maximum intensity. Pain is steady and moderate to very severe. There is little pain relief with changing position. Frequently, the pain is unbearable, steady, and boring. Bandlike radiation of the pain to the back occurs in half of the patients. Pain is absent in 5% to 10% of attacks, and a painless presentation may be a feature of serious fatal disease.

#### *Physical examination*

Physical findings vary with the severity of an attack. Patients with mild pancreatitis may not seem acutely ill. Abdominal tenderness may be mild, and abdominal guarding may be absent. In severe pancreatitis, patients look severely ill and often have abdominal distention, especially epigastric, which is due to gastric, small bowel, or colonic ileus. Almost all patients are tender in the upper abdomen, which may be elicited by gently shaking the abdomen or by gentle percussion. Guarding is more marked in the upper abdomen. Tenderness and guarding can be less than expected, considering the intensity of discomfort. Abdominal rigidity, as occurs in diffuse peritonitis, is unusual but can be present, and differentiation from a perforated viscus may be impossible in these instances. Bowel sounds are reduced and may be absent. Additional abdominal findings may include ecchymosis in 1 or both flanks (Grey Turner sign) or about the periumbilical area (Cullen sign) owing to extravasation of hemorrhagic pancreatic exudate to these areas. These signs occur in less than 1% of cases and are associated with a poor prognosis. The general examination, particularly in severe pancreatitis, may uncover markedly abnormal vital signs if there are third-space fluid losses and systemic toxicity. Commonly, the pulse rate is 100 to 150 beats per minute. Blood pressure can be initially higher than normal (perhaps because of pain) and then lower than normal with third-space losses and hypovolemia. Initially, the temperature may be normal, but within 1 to 3 days it may increase to 101° F to 103° F owing to the severe retroperitoneal inflammatory process and to the release of inflammatory mediators from the pancreas. Tachypnea with shallow respirations may be present if the subdiaphragmatic inflammatory exudate causes painful breathing. Dyspnea may accompany pleural effusions, atelectasis, acute respiratory distress syndrome (ARDS), or congestive heart failure. Chest examination may reveal limited diaphragmatic excursion if abdominal pain causes splinting of the diaphragm, or dullness to percussion and decreased breath sounds at the lung bases if there is a pleural effusion. There may be disorientation, hallucinations, agitation, or coma, which may be due to alcohol withdrawal, hypotension, fever, or toxic effects of pancreatic enzymes on the central nervous system. Conjunctival icterus, if present, may be due to choledocholithisis (gallstone pancreatitis) or bile duct obstruction from edema of the head of the pancreas, or from coexistent liver disease.

The differential diagnosis of acute pancreatitis is outlined in **Box 2**. The pain of perforated peptic ulcer is sudden, becomes diffuse, and precipitates a rigid abdomen; movement aggravates pain. In mesenteric ischemia or infarction, the clinical setting often is an older person with atrial fibrillation or arteriosclerotic disease who develops sudden pain out of proportion to physical findings, bloody diarrhea, nausea, and vomiting. In intestinal obstruction, pain is cyclical; abdominal distention is prominent; vomiting persists and may become feculent, and peristalsis is hyperactive and often audible.

- Laboratory Diagnosis
- Pancreatic enzymes
  - Amylase
  - Lipase
  - Other pancreatic enzyme levels
- Standard blood tests
- Diagnostic imaging
- Abdominal plain film
- Chest radiography
- Abdominal ultrasound
- Endoscopic ultrasound
- Endoscopic retrograde cholangiopancreatography (ERCP)
- CT
- MRI

## PHARMACOLOGIC TREATMENT OPTIONS

### *Management*

Patients with acute pancreatitis require early aggressive intravenous (IV) hydration to maintain hemodynamic stability and adequately perfuse the kidneys and pancreas (**Fig. 3**). Patients also need adequate analgesia to eliminate or markedly reduce pain. The patient is usually NPO (nothing by mouth) until any nausea and vomiting have subsided. Nastrogastric intubation is not used routinely because it is not

**Box 2**
**Differential diagnosis**

Biliary colic

Acute cholecystitis

Perforated hollow viscus (eg, perforated peptic ulcer)

Mesenteric ischemia or infarction

Intestinal obstruction

Myocardial infarction

Dissecting aortic aneurysm

Ectopic pregnancy

*From* Tenner S, Steinberg WM. Acute pancreatitis. In: Feldman M, Friedman LS, Brandt LJ, eds. Sleisenger and Fordtran's gastrointestinal and liver disease pathophysiology, diagnosis, management. 10th edition. Philadelphia: Elsevier; 2016; with permission.

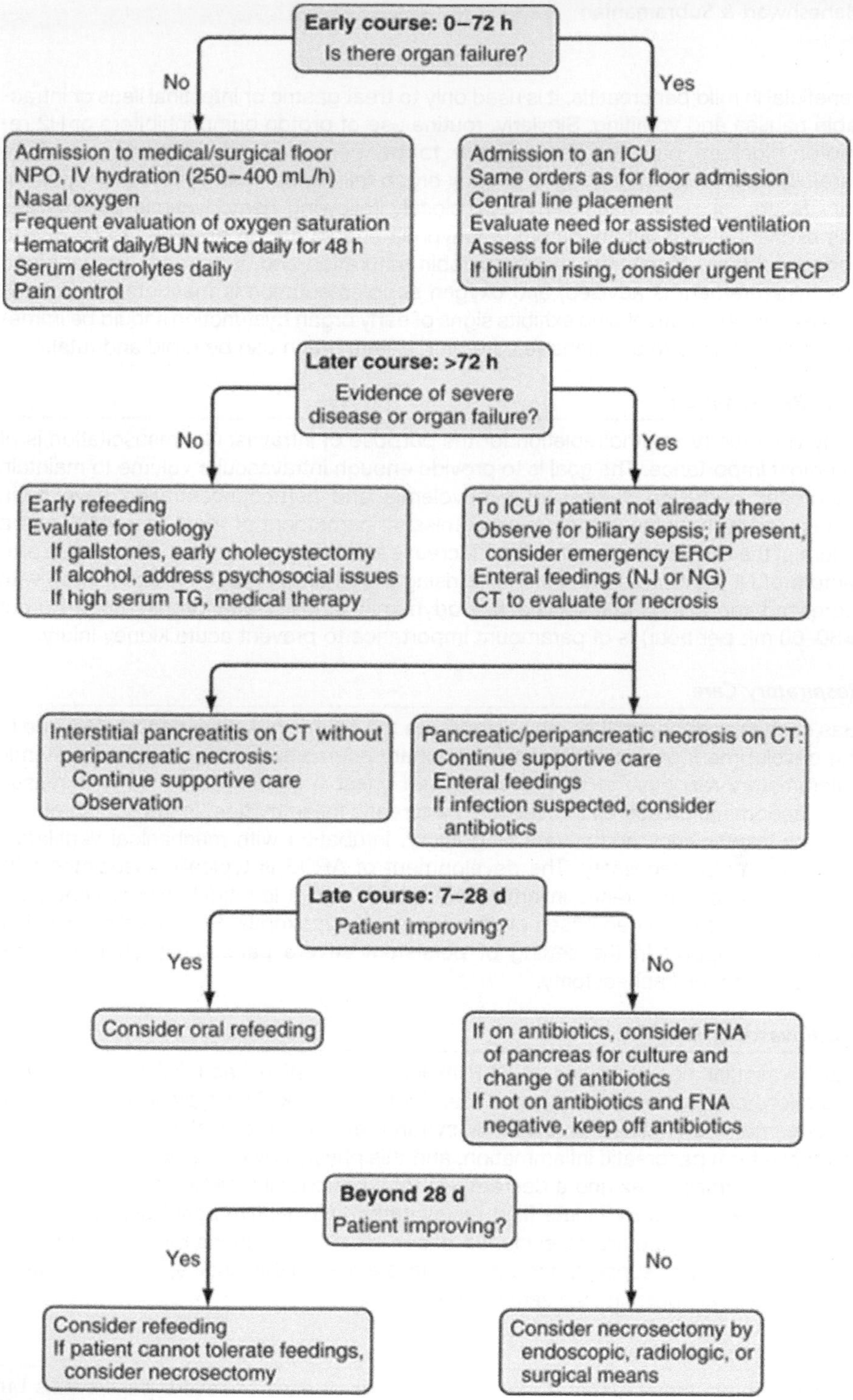


**Fig. 3.** Algorithm for the management of acute pancreatitis at various stages in its course. BUN, blood urea nitrogen; ICU, intensive care unit; NG, nasogastric; NJ, nasojejunal; TG, thyroglobulin. (*From* Tenner S, Steinberg WM. Acute pancreatitis. In: Feldman M, Friedman LS, Brandt LJ, eds. Sleisenger and Fordtran's gastrointestinal and liver disease pathophysiology, diagnosis, management. 10th edition. Philadelphia: Elsevier; 2016; with permission.)

beneficial in mild pancreatitis. It is used only to treat gastric or intestinal ileus or intractable nausea and vomiting. Similarly, routine use of proton pump inhibitors or H2 receptor blockers has not been shown to be beneficial. The patient should be carefully monitored for any signs of early organ failure, such as hypotension, pulmonary failure, or renal insufficiency, by closely following hemodynamic parameters, gas exchange, and urinary output. Tachypnea should not be assumed to be due to abdominal pain. Monitoring oxyhemoglobin saturation and, if needed, arterial blood gas measurement is advised, and oxygen supplementation is mandatory if there is hypoxemia. Any patient who exhibits signs of early organ dysfunction should be immediately transferred to an intensive care unit; deterioration can be rapid and fatal.

### *Fluid Resuscitation*

Early vigorous IV volume repletion for the purpose of intravascular resuscitation is of foremost importance. The goal is to provide enough intravascular volume to maintain pancreatic perfusion. Indices of hypovolemia and hemoconcentration have been associated with worse outcome; an admission hematocrit of more than 44% and a failure of the admission hematocrit to decrease at 24 hours have been show to be predictors of NP, and an elevation and/or rising blood urea nitrogen is associated with increased mortality.[6] Maintaining hemodynamic stability and proper urine output (>30–60 mL per hour) is of paramount importance to prevent acute kidney injury.

### *Respiratory Care*

Gas exchange abnormalities may complicate the course of severe pancreatitis due to the development of noncardiogenic pulmonary edema secondary due to a systemic inflammatory response or due to decreased chest wall compliance from increased intra-abdominal pressures from severe pancreatic inflammation. In the setting of pulmonary insufficiency and severe lung injury, intubation with mechanical ventilatory support may be necessary. The development of ARDS is typically associated with an extrathoracic pancreatic inflammatory cause, and a low tidal volume ventilatory strategy may be required based on the degree of hypoxemia. Prolonged mechanical ventilatory support in the setting of persistent severe pancreatitis should trigger consideration for tracheostomy.

### *Cardiovascular Care*

Cardiovascular complications of SAP include congestive heart failure, myocardial infarction, cardiac dysrhythmia, and cardiogenic shock. The typical hemodynamic derangement is a distributive shock syndrome due to a systemic inflammatory response from pancreatic inflammation, and this physiology is characterized by an increase in cardiac index and a decrease in total peripheral resistance. If hypotension persists even with appropriate fluid resuscitation, vasoactive agent support is indicated. Although there are no evidence-based recommendations for an initial choice of vasoactive agent support, norepinephrine is a reasonable choice, with the addition of low-dose vasopressin as a second agent.

### *Metabolic Complications*

Hyperglycemia may present during the first several days of severe pancreatitis but usually disappears as the inflammatory process subsides. Blood sugars fluctuate, and insulin should be administered cautiously. Hypocalcemia is almost uniformly present because of a low serum albumin. Because this calcium low is nonionized, hypocalcemia is largely asymptomatic and requires no specific therapy. However, reduced serum ionized calcium may occur and cause neuromuscular irritability. If hypomagnesemia coexists, magnesium replacement should restore serum calcium to normal.

### *Infectious Disease and Antibiotics*

In the absence of infection, antibiotics are not indicated in mild pancreatitis. However, antibiotics would be appropriate in pancreatic sepsis (eg, infected necrosis and, less often, abscess) and nonpancreatic sepsis (eg, line sepsis, urosepsis, or pneumonia). These septic conditions are major sources of morbidity and mortality in patients with SAP, and clinicians should be aware that these infectious complications account for many early and late deaths from the disease. Imipenem, fluoroquinolones (ciprofloxacin, ofloxacin, pefloxacin), and metronidazole are the drugs that achieve the highest inhibitory concentrations in pancreatic tissue, whereas aminoglycosides do not. Based on the latest 2 placebo-controlled studies, routine use of antibiotics is questionable in the absence of biliary sepsis or obvious pancreatic or peripancreatic infection.[6] Although previous practice guidelines recommend the use of prophylactic antibiotics in patients with severe NP, more recent reviews and guidelines state that prophylactic antibiotics should not be used for the purpose of preventing infection in patients with NP.[6] Infection of necrosis typically occurs after the 10th day of hospitalization. Infection of the pancreatic necrosis is thought to occur from translocation of bacteria from the colon. This finding may help explain why enteral feeding, decreasing the pathogenic intestinal flora, prevents infection of the necrosis. When infection is suspected, the diagnosis is readily established by CT-guided fine-needle aspiration (FNA). The procedure is safe and effective in establishing the diagnosis. The Gram stain alone has a sensitivity of almost 95% if carefully examined in a fresh specimen. The procedure is also safe, rarely introducing infection into a sterile field in the abdomen. If negative, an aspiration can be repeated every 4 to 7 days if infection continues to be suspected. In the past, the diagnosis of infected necrosis implied the urgent need for surgical debridement, but this is no longer always the case.

## NONPHARMACOLOGIC TREATMENT OPTIONS

### *Endoscopy*

The question of early removal of a possibly impacted gallstone in improving the outcome of gallstone pancreatitis remains a controversial issue. There is a consensus that severe acute gallstone pancreatitis with ascending cholangitis (jaundice and fever) is an indication for urgent ERCP. Until randomized studies are performed, it is not clear whether potential advantages of early pancreatic duct stenting outweigh the risks.

### *Nutrition*

Patients with SAP, especially with pancreatic necrosis, may need 4 to 6 weeks of artificial nutrition support. Formerly, total parenteral nutrition was the standard of care for feeding patients with SAP. Because enteral nutrition can stimulate pancreatic and intestinal secretions, the pancreatic rest concept has been a dogma in managing severe acute pancreatitis. However, bowel rest is associated with intestinal atrophy and bacterial overgrowth and is responsible for elevated endotoxin and cytokines levels, bacterial translocation, and systemic inflammatory response syndrome induction and is associated with a higher risk of infected pancreatic necrosis. Therefore, because of its beneficial effects on tissue of the intestinal mucosa and the splanchnic blood flow, the concept that enteral nutrition "worsens" pancreatitis has diminished greatly over recent years. In a recent meta-analysis including 8 randomized controlled studies and 381 patients, enteral nutrition compared with parenteral nutrition decreased infectious complications and mortality.[8] The use of early enteral nutrition (within 48 hours of admission) has proven to be beneficial in patients with acute pancreatitis because it improves clinical outcomes by reducing the number of infections, particularly pancreatic infections.[9] On the basis of the assumption that gastric food administration increases the risk of abdominal pain exacerbation, nasojejunal feeding has long been favored. However, exclusive gastric feeding succeeds with the delivery of nutritional targets in 90% of patients.[10]

## RADIOLOGIC AND SURGICAL TREATMENT OPTIONS

Cholecystectomy is routinely performed with gallstone pancreatitis, and a consensus conference suggested that in mild or severe gallstone pancreatitis, cholecystectomy should be performed as soon as the patient has recovered and the acute inflammatory process has subsided. A second potential role for surgery in pancreatitis is to debride pancreatic necrosis (necrosectomy) or drain a pancreatic abscess.[6]

Some investigators have reported that it is important to differentiate sterile necrosis from infected necrosis by FNA of the pancreas. Sterile necrosis can be managed nonoperatively because the mortality of this condition without surgery is less than 5%. On the other hand, infected necrosis (as documented by FNA of the pancreas with Gram stain and cultures) has been historically regarded as an indication for surgical debridement because of the previous thinking that infected necrosis treated medically has a nearly uniform fatal outcome. Surgical debridement of sterile pancreatic necrosis has also been shown not to be helpful in the vast majority of cases. Early surgical debridement is exceedingly difficulty and avoided within the first 4 to 8 days because of the cementlike nature of the necrosis.

Currently, the management of NP has undergone a paradigm shift toward minimally invasive techniques for necrosectomy, obviating open necrosectomy in most cases.[11] There is increasing evidence that minimally invasive approaches, including a step-up approach that incorporates percutaneous catheter or endoscopic transluminal drainage followed by video-assisted retroperitoneal or endoscopic debridement,[12] are associated with improved outcomes over traditional open necrosectomy for patients with infected NP. A recent international multidisciplinary consensus conference emphasized the superiority of minimally invasive approaches over standard surgical approaches.[3]

However, in a stable patient with infected necrosis, maximal supportive care and the use of pancreatic-penetrating antibiotics such fluoroquinolones, metronidazole, and imipenem or meropenem should be administered. Antibiotics have been shown to successfully treat infection of necrosis in many patients so it is possible that no other intervention will be needed. Even if intervention is needed owing to persistent symptoms, the antibiotics will allow time for the formation of a fibrous wall, creating WON. This fibrous wall assists in a successful minimally invasive approach to draining the pancreatic necrosis. Although early debridement of pancreatic necrosis within the first 4 to 5 weeks of an attack will require surgery, WON can be treated laparoscopically, percutaneously, or endoscopically. The timing and method of debridement require a clear discussion between the surgeon, gastroenterologist, and interventional radiologist, but should be left at the discretion of the pancreatic surgeon.

## EVALUATION OF OUTCOME AND LONG-TERM RECOMMENDATIONS

For sterile NP, the mortality of conservative treatment remained between 0% and 15.3%, which is the same as reported before 2000. Despite some studies' reports of single-digit mortality using surgical necrosectomy, high mortality (20.0%–63.9%) is reported in most series. Except in a few centers, surgical outcome has not changed much, and the surgical risk is high. A nationwide study in the United States of 1783 patients from 1998 to 2010 indicated that the incidence of pancreatic debridement significantly decreased from 0.44% to 0.25% and that in-hospital mortality (overall 22.0%) significantly decreased from 29.0% to 15%. Minimally invasive necrosectomy, mainly transluminal endoscopic necrosectomy with drainage, has shown remarkable results combined with percutaneous drainage (PCD) or using a metallic stent. The success rate of PCD varies. Some series report that it remains unchanged at 35% to 49%, but most have reached a higher success rate of 76% to 93%. The transluminal endoscopic drainage rates are about 80%, and even 100% when using single transluminal gateway transcystic multiple drainage methods. Single-digit mortality was reported in most series, and zero mortality is a reality.[13]

## SUMMARY

Acute pancreatitis varies widely in its clinical presentation, from clinically negligible to precipitously fatal despite any intervention. Progression to multiorgan failure can occur rapidly and portends a life-threatening course. NP is a manifestation of SAP associated with significant morbidity and mortality. The extent of necrosis correlates well with the incidence of infected necrosis, organ failure, need for debridement, and morbidity and mortality. Having established the diagnosis of pancreatic necrosis, goals of appropriately aggressive resuscitation should be established and adhered to in a multidisciplinary approach involving medical and surgical intensive care. Intervention for infected pancreatic necrosis should be based on a minimally invasive approach. In all cases of NP, a multidisciplinary approach is needed, using endoscopic techniques and/or PCD. Open surgery should be reserved for failure of less invasive techniques.

## REFERENCES

1. Fagenholz PJ, Fernández-del Castillo C, Harris NS, et al. Direct medical costs of acute pancreatitis hospitalizations in the United States. Pancreas 2007;35(4):302–7.
2. Lowenfels AB, Maisonneuve P, Sullivan T. The changing character of acute pancreatitis: epidemiology, etiology, and prognosis. Curr Gastroenterol Rep 2009;11(2):97–103.
3. Freeman ML, Werner J, van Santvoort HC, et al. Interventions for necrotizing pancreatitis: summary of a multidisciplinary consensus conference. Pancreas 2012;41(8):1176–94.
4. Haney JC, Pappas TN. Necrotizing pancreatitis: diagnosis and management. Surg Clin North Am 2007;87(6):1431–46, ix.
5. Hughes SJ, Papachristou GI, Federle MP, et al. Necrotizing pancreatitis. Gastroenterol Clin North Am 2007;36(2):313–23, viii.
6. Feldman M, Friedman LS, Brandt LJ, et al. Sleisenger and Fordtran's gastrointestinal and liver disease: pathophysiology, diagnosis, management. 10th edition. Philadelphia: Saunders/Elsevier; 2015.
7. Sabo A, Goussous N, Sardana N, et al. Necrotizing pancreatitis: a review of multidisciplinary management. JOP 2015;16(2):125–35.
8. Yi F, Ge L, Zhao J, et al. Meta-analysis: total parenteral nutrition versus total enteral nutrition in predicted severe acute pancreatitis. Intern Med 2012;51(6):523–30.

9. Li JY, Yu T, Chen GC, et al. Enteral nutrition within 48 hours of admission improves clinical outcomes of acute pancreatitis by reducing complications: a meta-analysis. PLoS One 2013;8(6):e64926.
10. Nally DM, Kelly EG, Clarke M, et al. Nasogastric nutrition is efficacious in severe acute pancreatitis: a systematic review and meta-analysis. Br J Nutr 2014; 112(11):1769–78.
11. Trikudanathan G, Arain M, Attam R, et al. Interventions for necrotizing pancreatitis: an overview of current approaches. Expert Rev Gastroenterol Hepatol 2013;7(5):463–75.
12. van Santvoort HC, Besselink MG, Bakker OJ, et al. A step-up approach or open necrosectomy for necrotizing pancreatitis. N Engl J Med 2010;362(16):1491–502.
13. Chang YC. Is necrosectomy obsolete for infected necrotizing pancreatitis? Is a paradigm shift needed? World J Gastroenterol 2014;20(45):16925–34.

# Index

*Note:* Page numbers of article titles are in **boldface** type.




Crit Care Clin 32 (2016) 291–299
http://dx.doi.org/10.1016/S0749-0704(16)30009-4
criticalcare.theclinics.com

I



L

Printed and bound by CPI Group (UK) Ltd, Croydon, CR0 4YY
03/10/2024
01040388-0011